Getting Pregnant with Ease

Sustainable Life Choices for Improved Fertility

Chika Samuels

Getting Pregnant with Ease

Copyright © 2020 by **Chika Samuels**

ISBN: 978-978-978-904-7

Published in Nigeria by:
Cgnature Creativemedia Ltd.
19, Mabinuori Street, off Association Road
Shangisha, Near Magodo Ph 2, Lagos.
t: +234.708.684.2032
e: cgnaturestudio@gmail.com

For more information on this book or to order, visit
http://www.soprecious.ng/fertilitybook

For more information about the author and additional products, programmes and partnership opportunities,
visit, www.soprecious.ng
email us, info@soprecious.ng
call us, +2348062808307

Printed in Nigeria

Dedication

This book is dedicated to the bravest woman that ever lived – Mrs Rose Obioma Okoh. Many say she was my mother-in-law but to her, I was the epitome of perfection and she showed it to the world in every way possible.

May her sweet soul continue to rest in the bosom of our Lord.

Amen.

Acknowledgements

My deep appreciation goes to the Lord Almighty who guided my heart towards putting my experience, journey and thoughts on paper so that it may be imprinted on the sands of time, granted me the ability to be an inspiration to many around the world and helped me choose the correct lifestyle for wellness and good living – just the way He created us to function!

To my husband, the man of my dreams: Your kind heart, enduring tolerance, consistent support and lavish show of love are rare in our world today and I do not take these for granted.

To my family & friends: Thank you for standing by me through all seasons of life.

To all intending mothers, who have shared their problems and feelings with me, who have taught me more than any book could: Thank you for giving me the privilege to build a family with you.

To those who yearn to have a child of their own; I look forward to archiving your little one's picture on our SoPrecious Wall of Miracles gallery.

Who this Book is For

1. Every wo(man) that has been trying to conceive for more than 2 years or has previously experienced a miscarriage.

2. Every wo(man) between the ages of 18 and 45.

3. Every woman that intends to birth or nurse a child.

4. Every bride (groom)-to-be

5. Every urban wo(man).

6. Every man who wants improved health for procreation.

7. Those who desire to have more children

8. Those interested in Pre-menopausal health care.

9. Everyone interested in improving their overall vitality & health, as well as adopting sustainable healthy lifestyle habits.

If you have a loved one who is struggling with infertility, a gift of this book is the best thing you can do for them.

Contents

viii

Foreword

Infertility is "*a disease of the reproductive system defined by the failure to achieve a clinical pregnancy after 12 months or more of regular unprotected sexual intercourse*"...WHO-ICMART-AFS-ASRM-ESHRE-ASPIRE.

One in four couples experiences infertility in developing countries. And it has shown an almost similar prevalence worldwide due to improved technology, late marriages, increased consumption of highly processed foods, environmental toxins, and a host of other changes our world today is experiencing.

As a reproductive endocrinologist/IVF consultant for over four decades and I have seen couples or intending parents walk into my office for support in assisted reproduction- most times, after which they have seemingly exhausted all options of natural conception. We seem to have forgotten about ourselves being the most important when it comes to reproduction, and we tend to chase something outside ourselves for that to happen. How better would our world be if we could "self-rejuvenate" or "self-heal" our body system by simply adopting sustainable lifestyle habits? I have also discovered and resonate with Dr. Robert Morse N.D that there are no incurable diseases, only fatal people.

Chika took an honourable and selfless step to write a critical book such as this, to help other women with similar experiences

x

as herself in a society where exceptional knowledge is rare, and silence/ ignorance thrives amongst those in the quest for a child.

What's impressive about this book is that it gives evidence-based insights into critical factors that affect fertility and packed with tips, suggestions, tools, and practical techniques for gaining results in the complex world of infertility. It is an enthusiastic celebration of strength, patience, and commitment in its expedient manner that instantly springs its reader to action, to take their health into their hands, and play their roles to create the required changes in their body.

I have spent the last 20 years, improving the ability to conceive through the set-up of Modern Mayr Medicine to promote reproductive health. Chika's book complements that concept. I, therefore, recommend this book to those who have been trying to conceive. And to those who are interested in improving general well-being and vitality in an urban society such as ours. It is a must-have in your arsenal of alternative restorative measures.

Prof. Oladapo A Ashiru OFR
MB., BS; MS, PHD, FASN, FEMSON, HCLD/CC(ABB-USA)
PROFESSOR AND CONSULTANT REPRODUCTIVE ENDOCRINOLOGIST
CHIEF MEDICAL DIRECTOR
MEDICAL ART CENTER.

Statistics

For the purpose of this book, we shall adopt a definition of 'infertility' as set forth in the guidelines of the Royal College of Obstetricians and Gynaecologists (UK): "failure to conceive after regular sexual intercourse for two years in the absence of known reproductive pathology".Infertility is the most important reproductive health problem in developing countries, with the lifetime prevalence rate increasing from 6.6% to 32.6%. Infertility can affect one's whole life and it is associated with dysthymia, anxiety and more diseases. However, in most developing countries, reproductive health care is synonymous with family planning. Attention is given only to the decreasing number of births in these countries but infertility care is given little or no attention.[1]

Let's take Nigeria as a case study. The country has over 193 million people as at the beginning of 2018 (the number was around 190 million in 2017). Yet about 20-25 percent of local couples are childless. This 20-25 percent prevalence of infertility in Nigeria is for couples that are officially married. Still, these numbers could be higher as medical institutions report their own statistics. It is societally expected that a woman must give birth to her own children. Infertility between couples is generally ascribed to the female, albeit erroneously.

---

1. https://www.ncbi.nlm.nih.gov/pmc/articles/PMC3701979/

A study was carried out in one of the states In Nigeria, with a population of about 3.5 million (according to the last national population census). In the state, there are eight general hospitals, functional infertility clinics, two teaching hospitals, organized Obstetrics and Gynaecology departments with human resources to manage infertility in the state. The study was a descriptive cross-sectional survey among infertile women. A total of 250 respondents returned completely filled questionnaires, giving a response rate of 97.3%. The results revealed that the 25- 34 age group constitutes the highest (44.4%) amongst other age groups. One hundred and ninety (76.0%) of these respondents were married, 47.6% of respondents are skilled workers. This shows that a good percentage of women struggling with infertility **are *urban skilled working/ business married women***

One of the reliable studies[2] also reveals that the major cause of infertility in Nigeria is *infection:* sexually transmitted diseases (STDs), postabortal and puerperal sepsis, and these problems are by no means restricted to women. However, male infertility is regarded as taboo, a problem that no one will admit exists. This taboo itself is a contributor to practices of polygyny, with women all too frequently assumed by the local population to be the primary culprit in- infertile marriages, and male infertility handled with discretion, to protect male dignity.

This book considered previous studies in Nigeria which focused on the possible contributions of environmental factors, such

2. *A review of management of infertility in Nigeria: framing the ethics of a national health policy (https://www.ncbi.nlm.nih.gov/pmc/articles/PMC3163656/)*

as diet and toxic elements, sociocultural behaviours and socio-demographic factors, infections, and hormones. Another study also acknowledges that "irrespective of source, health care development in Nigeria is largely limited to curative services, with prevention, promotion, rehabilitation and other aspects *receiving attention only on paper*".[3] Infertility as a problem faces stiff competition for available resources in this context. Given that "current health spending in most low-income countries is insufficient for the achievement of the health MDGs,"[4] it is debatable that infertility reasonably has a place in public sector financing, though it has a place in privately financed options via established fertility intervention units like SoPrecious Fertility Intervention Centres.

In the case of Nigeria, this would include an increase in per capita expenditure within the health system from US$9.44 to US$34 as recommended by the WHO. Of course, as former WHO Director-General, Dr Lee Jong-wook, conceded, "The MDGs do not say everything that needs to be said about health and development" – and he specifically mentioned reproductive health as one of the needs not included in the MDGs. The data showed that urban women in Nigeria do not desire to stop childbearing until they have reached an advanced age and have a relatively large number of children. These findings are reflective of a high fertility setting where

3. (Alubo O, Health Policy Plan, Danis M, Sepinwall A, The Promise and Limits of Private Medicine: Health Policy Dilemmas in Nigeria. J Law Med Ethics. 2002 Winter; 30(4):667-76. [PubMed] [Ref list], Regulation of the Global Marketplace for the Sake of Health)

4. Disease Control Priorities in Developing Countries. 2nd edition. Top of Form Millennium Development Goals for Health: What Will It Take to Accelerate Progress? By Adam Wagstaff, Mariam Claeson, Robert M. Hecht, Pablo (https://www.ncbi.nlm.nih.gov/books/NBK11716/)

pro-natalist attitudes are prevalent and are reminiscent of what other studies in Nigeria have suggested.[5]These studies and more reveal that most causes of maternal deaths can be prevented by improved management of pregnancy-related complications. Maternal nutrition plays a crucial role in influencing fertility, fetal development, birth outcomes, and breast milk composition. During the critical window of time from conception through the initiation of complementary feeding, the nutrition of the mother is the nutrition of the offspring – and a mother's dietary and lifestyle choices can affect both the early health status and lifelong disease risk of the offspring.

This is the exact gap that this book intends to fill, helping intending parents create as many healthy babies as they desire, when they desire. We will guide you from conception till you hold a health baby in your arms.

What this Book Offers You

Getting Pregnant with Ease is a lifestyle and fertility guide and will help you get in the best possible shape before you even start trying to get pregnant- to maximize your chances of conceiving quickly. The intent of this book is not just to help you get pregnant but to help you nurture a healthy baby and enjoy a wholesome post-partum stage. This book takes a spirit-mind-body approach that will help identify and address the spiritual, mental, emotional and physical factors which affect fertility and reduce the negative effects of infertility. It

---

5. *https://www.who.int/reproductivehealth/publications/monitoring/maternal-mortality-2015/en/*

will give you evidence-based insight to critical factors that affect fertility and is packed with tips, suggestions, tools and practical techniques for gaining results with each stage of fertility intervention.

If you're concerned that you might have problems conceiving –or if you've been trying for more than two years – *Getting Pregnant with Ease* will give you the comprehensive information you need in your quest for a child. It will also help you and your partner navigate the complex worlds of fertility and infertility. In this guide, we explore the pros and cons of several dietary theories to help each individual find their optimal way of eating and living. This book will zoom in on "primary food", which is what I tag the 3 cardinal areas of your life. Primary food, by our definition goes beyond what is on your plate. Your primary food is all that your skin absorbs, your mouth takes in, your thought processes and the meditations of your heart.

Your primary food comprises healthy relationships (with self, family, community), the right nourishment, regular physical activity, a fulfilling career, a spiritual practice and effective mind management. These can fill your soul and satisfy your hunger for life. Trust me, when your primary food is balanced and satiating, your life feeds you, making what you eat secondary.

By reading this fertility guide, you will:

- Get pregnant fast! If you consistently apply the principles within this book, you will get into a state where procreating will come easily.

- Get connected to a rich and active support community of women from all walks of life with a singular purpose of living life with full blast and blessing the world with healthy babies.

- Access a comprehensive list of useful resources that deal with the medical, emotional, and other aspects of fertility.

- Become more aware of what is going on in your body, why you feel or act the way you do and how all these impact your fertility – body literacy.

- Be empowered to take your fertility into your hands and create the required changes to progress in your life goals.

How to Use this Book for Best Outcomes

If you have been diagnosed with specific conditions that affect your fertility, your natural inclination may be to flip through and turn directly to the chapters that deal with your particular problem. To get the most from this book, you need to know the basics of each principle so you can correctly apply the suggestions contained in the book's later chapters. If you give attention to *each* page, you will be able to understand the causes of your own particular fertility challenges and then discover how to treat them using ancient forms of self-healing. Nutritional habits and routines often need consistency for full recovery to take place. Making changes in what, when, and how we eat and drink, as well as adding certain forms of exercise, massages, affirmation, meditation, and other self-care techniques, can contribute significantly to enhancing your fertility.

A Chinese proverb states: "When the soil is well prepared, the harvest will be bountiful." Any gardener will tell you that the quality of the soil is what influences the productivity and health of the plant. Preparing the soil isn't the most glamorous job: it takes time to turn the soil and balance the pH, and if done naturally, it can involve smelly things like manure and compost. In the same way, changing our diet and lifestyle can at times be unglamorous. We have to say no to some addictions such as coffee or refined sugar or even excess worry. We may have to make some sacrifices by giving up certain habits that may be delaying conception or disrupting it's cycle. We have to change some household items that are hormone disruptors. We may have to skip the convenience of fast food, using microwave and prepare your own home-made healthful food instead. We may have to forsake a couple of hours of TV to spend time doing our faith practices, meditating or exercising. Like they say, "something has got to give".

One thing is sure: as you apply every recommendation religiously, you will find that these lifestyle changes offer you two compensations. First, you will discover a much greater feeling of health and vitality within yourself when you start really taking care of the needs of your body, mind, and spirit. Second, you can be certain that you are doing everything possible to prepare the first and most important "home" for your future child- which is your own body! Please note that this book is not a fertility quick fix or a one-size-fits-all remedy; restoring the body to health takes time. If you are reading this book and wish to apply to your own condition, you must give yourself at least three months for the interventions to have full effect.

As you interact with our website *(www.soprecious.ng)*, you will see links to our community where you will need to engage our fertility experts and partner medical practitioners, take some quizzes so we can get clearer understanding of your case, carry out some exercises (like the *#SoPreciousfertilitydare*), utilise critical recommendations like our 17-week Prior-conception Programme , One-on-one coaching sessions or Conception Cycle Demystified Programme, etc. The good news is, you don't have to wait too long to get tangible physical results! Over the first few weeks of applying the principles here, you should look for specific changes, some of which may occur quickly. Are your symptoms improving? Are your breasts less tender at ovulation? Are your cycles becoming more regular? Is your flow better? Are you experiencing fewer mood swings before menstruation? Whatever your symptoms are, you should experience improvement in them as your body restores itself to hormonal health.

Also, remember that some conditions have been a long time in the making, and it may take a while for the body to unmake them. Give your body time; use how you feel to gauge your progress with the programme. Are you feeling healthier? More normal hormonally? Is your reproductive system starting to respond as it's supposed to during the course of a monthly cycle? Use your subjective response as your most accurate gauge. Renowned fertility experts have claimed that pregnancy comes when certain symptoms either appear or disappear. Give your body a chance to heal itself, and watch out for progress.

Introduction

Whether this is your second, or fifth or tenth year of trying to conceive, I am super excited and tremendously honoured to share this journey with you and most thrilled to be your guide on this transformative expedition. All that you will learn in this book falls into the category of **transformational change, if you choose** to *diligently* and *consistently* implement what you learn here and in our community.

Along this journey you and I are set to begin, you must set aside age, infertility complications, sperm abnormalities, medical reports, miscarriages, failed IVFs. No matter what your unique situation is today, the valuable principles in this book promise a solution. My charge to you today is to give this a chance and dare to be fully committed to the recommendations.

Our effective methodology cuts across 3 main stages of intervention:

1. The prior-conception preparation;

2. The conception attempt and

3. The post-pregnancy stage – for optimum results.

xx

The SoPrecious Approach to Fertility

SoPrecious fertility interventions adopt a set of holistic support steps that focus on nourishing food and lifestyle choices that addresses root causes of fertility issues. We emphasise the importance of local and organic produce, whole grains, high-quality animal proteins, healthy plant-based fats, and water. Healing for fertility must happen at the cellular level for true, lasting health and vitality to exist. All life, no matter how small or how large (atoms to universes and everything in between), when manifested physically, must have a mental body (mind portion) and an emotional body (astral portion).

Your cells respond to external stimuli not only from hormones, minerals, sugars, proteins and the like. The cell's ability to function is greatly affected by the body's pH factors (acidosis), congestion, types of foods consumed, and chemical consumption. Most people are not aware but your cells also respond to thoughts and emotions (feelings). The types of thoughts and feelings you have, harbour or carry around with you play a *major role* in cellular functioning. By extension, the wait time in your fertility journey can be affected by this. SoPrecious interventions encourage women to look at these aspects of life, which we refer to as "primary food" as a form of nourishment that can make life extraordinary.

The SoPrecious fertility and lifestyle interventions sessions are delivered in various facets e.g. One-on-One coaching sessions, Fertility focused group sessions, webinars etc.

The mode of delivery includes literature (books, blogs, social media contests) workshop-style webinars, transcripts and

xxi

Facebook Live sessions in a dedicated group, where you will have direct access to have your questions and get the answers you need to better understand your conception cycle, window of fertility and when to "get it done". This session demystifies the peculiarities of your cycle, recommends sustainable lifestyle changes and how to adapt easily to them, and provides strategies to improve liver function as this will be an important area to address to improve egg quality. By reading *Getting Pregnant with Ease*, you increase your chances of getting pregnant.

Once they make a decision to start a family, most couples think it will happen pretty quickly, if not the first time they have unprotected sex. The reality, however, is that it takes the average, healthy, young couple six months to a year to conceive. Age is an important fertility factor; the older you are, the longer it's likely to take you to conceive and have a successful pregnancy. Unfortunately, it will take many couples – even young, healthy ones – considerably longer than a year to conceive. Infertility – which is also quite common – is defined as the inability of a couple to achieve a successful pregnancy after one year of unprotected intercourse. A woman is considered infertile, therefore, if she has not become pregnant after a year of trying, and a man as infertile if he cannot father a child. This book aims to reduce "conception wait time" among the urban busy couples by educating them about body literacy and fertility awareness.

In working with numerous women trying to conceive, we have identified 3 key problems which all couples experience on their journey through infertility:

They don't know WHY they are not getting pregnant and this makes them curious and open to all manner of myths, junk information and fear.

They feel they have tried everything and all to no avail; this makes them very reluctant to try out new things and what seems similar to what they had tried before.

They are tired of "putting their life on hold" and just want to move on to the next stage of their life as a family as they intended from the beginning.

To resolve these frustrations, SoPrecious lifestyle and fertility interventions offer a proven, comprehensive methodology underpinned by a holistic and integrative intervention process, blending the best of natural and modern medicine to take home healthy babies. On the first day of our SoPrecious one-on-one fertility sessions, a client who has had multiple miscarriages said to me, "See, I have my own strategy of managing my health and lifestyle, I do not need to make all these lifestyle changes. There are people living with worse health conditions yet they are popping out babies." My response was, "Has your strategy worked? If it has not, why you don't give this a chance? At least, my strategies have produced results for other people."

There are people who quit before they even start. My first dare to you is: **DON'T BE THAT PERSON.**

Find your strength again, because when it comes to transforming your fertility, I can promise you there is light at the end of the tunnel. Take it from the woman who had the best doctors give the options of getting an egg donor, IVF or adopting a child – I am that woman! I will be sharing incredible values in mastering and applying simple choices to get you on your way to healthy babies. This book is designed as a proactive and applied learning tool and I am here, to guide your discovery, to encourage and inspire your commitment and support you. I expect you to dare to believe again, take charge of your fertility, your life, and your results.

CHAPTER 1

*"Any fertility intervention which is not cellular
in approach is nothing but a mirage."*

- Chika Samuels

IIIIIIIIIIIIIIIIIIIIIIIIIIIIIIIIIIIIIIIIIIIIIIIIIIIIIIIIIIIIIIIIIIIIIIIIIIIIIIIII

Fertility Awareness &
Defining Expectations

Who recalls the clay pots that our grannies would cook and
store food and water in? These were abandoned in favour
of storing in plastics, aluminium etc. Their foods, fruits and
vegetables were simple and so was their method of cooking
and preservation. Vegetables, seeds, herbs, spices and nuts
were their medicine, snacks and main meals. Now, we are
too urbanized and disregard these things that are nature's
blessings.

Urbanization, as fantastic as it is, has dealt horribly with our
bodies. While we consider it modern to eat processed food,

use microwaves and all sorts of plastics, the so-called "poor people" living in derelict situations cannot afford the urban life and so, their exposure to toxins, refrigeration, microwaving and plastics is minimal. This eventually has an impact on child-bearing and fertility. When your medical report for infertility gets complex, light should be thrown on your consumption. Let's go "cellular" on what we consume.

The pH value tells you if something is an acid, a base, or neutral.

A pH of 0 indicates a high level of acidity.

A pH of 7 is neutral.

A pH of 14 is the most basic, or alkaline.

For example, battery acid is extremely acidic at 0, while liquid drain cleaner is very alkaline at 14. Pure distilled water is in the middle at 7. It's neither acidic nor alkaline.

Just like different substances, different parts of the human body have different pH levels. For example, your ideal blood pH is between 7.35 and 7.45, which is slightly alkaline. The stomach is typically at a pH of 3.5, which helps food break down properly. Foods that are considered acidic have a pH level of 4.6 or lower. The following are some acidic foods that I trust may be found in your pantry or food store:

- Grains such as rice, wheat, etc.

- Sugar

- Flour products

- Certain dairy products

- Processed foods and meats, such as corned beef and sausages

- Sodas and other sweetened beverages

"What has PH got to do with my food?" you may ask.

When your diet is *predominantly* "acid forming", your hormones become out of balance, your food then ferments and putrefies instead of properly digesting. Excessive mucus and inflammation is produced. Your blood becomes toxic and your lymphatic system becomes clogged. This is what doctors diagnose as *disease* and manifests as the various inflammatory fertility illnesses we have like fibroids, etc. Inflammation can affect ovulation and hormone production, and can be associated with endometriosis. Inflammation is a major cause of infertility affecting essentially all components necessary for reproduction[1]. The SoPrecious approach to healing infertility is holistic and geared towards keeping your system alkaline, toxic free, and clean – internally, as well as externally.

Some reputable studies have confirmed that consistent changes in diet and lifestyle can greatly increase the likelihood of conception, proving that one can actually consume clean nutrients in forms that work well for the body's reproductive system as not all ingredients are created equal.

---

1. *https://www.ncbi.nlm.nih.gov/pmc/articles/PMC3107847/*

Goal Setting for Fertility

*"The laws of motion were not discovered
by the contemplation of inertia"*

— Chika Samuels —

I believe that when the mind and body are in a state of well-being, the body will naturally produce the conditions needed for reproduction. I dare say that equilibrium and well-being are an important aspect of fertility and reproduction. The woman's body was made to conceive, carry to term and bear healthy children. This is the truth and how God has made us to be and this is why I am passionate about helping every woman, who desires to be called "mum" by one who comes from her womb, have their dreams come through.

We know however, that millions of people get pregnant and have babies when they are mentally, emotionally and physically unwell, such as the mentally unstable women that give birth by the road side or someone who smokes or uses hard drugs yet gives birth to children- Let's not forget that each person's epigenetics predispositions are different, meaning the way each environmental factor impacts one person can be completely varied from how it impacts another. So, while some say that overall well-being may not be necessary for fertility, it certainly seems that improving well-being and restoring balance can enhance fertility and increase the chances of having a wholesome baby. Although it is possible to work directly with the known causes of fertility problems, there is still so much that is unknown about fertility and so working towards improving spiritual, psychological, and physical health is more likely to address the unknown causes tagged as "unexplainable infertility".

In helping women with "unexplainable or complex infertility", we have found that addressing the critical factors (which mostly are not identified by scans and general medical practitions by their doctors) are the game changer. In general terms, *a fertile state* is a state of mental, spiritual and physical balance which is experienced as a state of well-being. What this actually means to each individual will be an entirely unique thing. In order to understand what this means, you will need to answer a series of questions using the link on our website (www.soprecious.ng) that will lead you to take the SoPrecious Fertility Self-appraisal Scorecard. These questions are designed to get specific and detailed information about what it would be like for you to be in a fertile state. The self-appraisal score card is an essential part of the journey towards having your child(ren) in your arms. For intervention in any condition, the set goal is vitally important. This is one of the things we do on the first day of any of our fertility intervention session. Your goal needs to be clearly defined, realistic and achievable in order to guarantee success. A well-formed goal needs to be SMART and healthy. A SMART goal is one that is Specific, Measurable, Achievable, Realistic and Timely. A healthy goal is rational, flexible and consistent with reality.

Typically, when someone comes to see me with fertility concerns, they come with the implicit goal of having a baby. Certainly this is true in the majority of cases but there are, of course, those who come to see me with other additional goals, such as wanting a baby but not wanting to gain weight, or some are seeking relief from stress, seeking to quit smoking or drinking, wanting to stop worrying, needing to do away with plastic usage, overcoming phobia for childbirth or hospitals, overcoming hurt and unforgiveness, marital issues and so on. Although people often come with the sole motivation of having a baby, an important part of the healing process involves creating tailored goals in a SMART and healthy way, helping them recognise that the singular goal of having a baby might be counterproductive if not well-managed.

Confirmation of 100% commitment to our recommendations is one that is definite to tick on our intervention programmes. You must be willing to give the programme the desired attention. You cannot say you really want a baby but are not willing to *take immediate action* towards the recommendations. To aim to achieve something that ultimately may not happen (because of lack of 100% commitment) will lead to stress, anxiety, hopelessness and potential failure. It is important, therefore, to separate *the intention* from *the goal. An intention* is a hope and a desired outcome whereas *the goal* must be something that can be worked towards and achieved; it should help to make the couple's intention to have a baby far more likely. Making the distinction between the intention and the goal not only ensures that we are both working towards something that is obtainable but minimises the likelihood of false expectations, disappointment and further feelings of hopelessness.

Whose Problem is it, Anyway?

Infertility is a disease of numerous etiologies, which can affect both men and women of every ethnic group and race around the world. Though it is rarely considered a health issue of serious concern, infertility can lead to distress and depression, as well as discrimination and ostracism in certain cultures.[2] In the not-so-distant past, many people–even some doctors–assumed that infertility was entirely due to the woman. Although that assumption is still occasionally made today, there is increasing recognition that something may be amiss with the male partner as well. Indeed, in half of infertility cases, the man has a fertility problem. Infertility can be caused by a number of factors attributable to the man, the woman, or both. The man has the exclusive problem 30% of the time, and the couple has a combined problem 20% of the time.

The term "female factor" is used to describe conditions or disorders that contribute to infertility in women; while the term "male factor" is used to describe those that cause infertility in men. Individually, each factor may not impact greatly on your ability to conceive, but together, they throw the odds against you. For example, a woman who has a subtle cervical mucus problem might not have trouble conceiving if her partner has a normal sperm count. However, if her partner has a low sperm count, her chances of conceiving are greatly reduced. You get it now, right?

Let's consider Nigeria again as a case study. We invest so

---

2. https://www.ncbi.nlm.nih.gov/pmc/articles/PMC6757383/

much in big weddings, but after the excitement of wedding bells, the decision to start a family is barely made. So, when a woman begins to prepare for babies, she considers the relationship with her partner, her career goals, her biological clock, the size of their first home, the neighbourhood where they reside and the size of their savings account. However, there's one important issue that many couples tend to overlook, and that is the *state of their health*. The culture of routine health check ups that exists in developed nations is yet to catch on in developing countries, mostly because of poverty levels. Hence, the yardstick of how sexually active or abstinent she has been in her younger years, becomes the singular factor of consideration to judge if her body is ready for conception or not.

If you've been mostly healthy, there's probably no reason to think that this should be an issue when you decide to start a family. However, there is a lot you can and should do to be in the best state of health before trying to conceive- these are not things we are taught in schools. In our society, we frown at and do not discuss contraceptives, sex education and healthy sex communication at home or in schools, hence leaving social media and the internet to educate our little ones. Early awareness and education is one issue I hold close to my heart and hope to explore to educate and guide our growing generation aright concerning their sexuality, early lifestyle choices and body awareness so they can make the right choices even in the toughest times of their young lives.

The stigma associated with infertility makes many intending couples who struggle with infertility to turn to the internet(online sources) for information. While the internet can be an excellent medium for disseminating reproductive health information, quality reviews of fertility websites have demonstrated that this information may not be wholly accurate or accessible.[3] An Upsala Journal of medical sciences study published two articles in June 2018 - "What do people know about fertility?" and "A systematic review on fertility awareness and its associated factors -Perception of infertility and acceptability of assisted reproduction technology in northern Nigeria" and found that fertility awareness among reproductive-age people is low to moderate, even though awareness regarding the remaining risk factors was generally high. Two exceptions were two studies from Nigeria and Ukraine, which found low awareness regarding STIs (Sexually transmitted diseases). These results might be related to cultural and content differences regarding sexual education curricula. This difference is particularly relevant because STIs are responsible for a higher proportion of fertility problems in developing countries, both in women and men.

Being in the best shape to procreate involves more than just being free from disease; it includes such factors as eating the right foods, maintaining a healthy weight, being physically active, etc. It also involves being free from sexually transmitted diseases (STDs), which are more common than most people suspect. While most couples certainly know what's normally involved in getting pregnant, they often

3. Internet use and stigmatized illness. Berger M, Wagner TH, Baker LC Soc Sci Med. 2005 Oct; 61(8):1821-7.

don't know what they can do to maximise their chances of success of having a healthy baby. This is what we address during the days of the 7-day SoPrecious Fertility Dare. There's a saying that goes, "There is no way to describe light to a blind man". You do not know what you do not know and what you do not know may be what is standing between you and carrying a healthy baby to term and delivering safely. One thing is certain: There's a lot more to making babies than making love!

The Preconception Checkup

"Control is in view and possible when you know exactly what you are dealing with."

— Chika Samuels —

The main purpose of a preconception exam is to rule out diseases that can interfere with your chances of conceiving and carrying a healthy baby to full term. Although the woman is the one who becomes pregnant and gives birth, both parents can pass on genetic disorders. Men must ensure that they too, are healthy because medical conditions, both past and present, affect the development of sperm and their ability to fertilize eggs and produce a healthy embryo. It's important for both partners to be aware of the medical issues related to conception, pregnancy, and childbearing. When I meet with intending mothers and ask how long they have been trying to conceive for, they typically say anything between 2-9 years. My next question usually is, "Have both of you seen a doctor?" and often times, the answer is "Emm, not really."

Hey Mom, you need to know _exactly_ what you are dealing with. Even if you are exercising your faith for the child, It is critical that you know exactly what you are up against. For instance, If you haven't gotten pregnant within six months of unprotected sexual intercourse then your male partner should go for a semen analysis. Although this will ultimately have to be done and even repeated several times, doing it early can save time and even needless testing and intervention. Many women have gone through years of expensive, invasive infertility interventions only later to discover that their partners have low sperm counts/motility. (Keep in mind that even if a man has fathered a child in the past, his semen can change over time; he should still go for a semen analysis.)

Just because your test results fall within expected ranges does not make them optimal for fertility, I always emphasise that there is a huge difference between optimal health and optimal fertility; some things may be permissible for others in their healthy living pursuits but inadequate or not acceptable in the path of optimal health. For example, because of ray sensitivities to embryo, I often recommend a Hystero Contrast Sonography (HYCOSY) over the Hysterosalpingography (HSG) to avoid your reproductive organs being exposed to radiation and dyes. Another good example is the use of plastics for food storage in extreme temperatures- this may fly for people who are not procreating anymore but is a 'no-no' for optimal fertility.

If you're at all concerned that you might have a fertility problem, start by make an appointment by using link on our website (www.soprecious.ng) below to book a session with us.

What can Conceivably go Wrong

Disease is not the presence of something evil, but rather the lack of the presence of something essential.

— Dr. Bernard Jensen —

Successful conception and pregnancy depends on many factors, Some of these factors can interfere with a woman's ability to ovulate, conceive, or even carry a pregnancy to term; other factors can adversely affect a man's ability to produce *viable* sperm and deliver the sperm into a woman's vagina. And to further complicate things, each partner can have multiple problems. For example, an irregular cycle is a simple sign of an imbalance in the hormones and this is the gap that our "SoPrecious Conception Cycle Demystified" programme fills. Fertility problems are in different categories; nothing with regard to reproduction is that simple or straightforward.

 Most people choose to eat a predominantly acid-forming diet, and as a result, over-acidic (acidosis) conditions of the body (both systemic and cellular) begin to take place. *Acidosis* and *inflammation* are virtually the same thing, just different terminologies. Added to these acidic diets are the acid-type hormones. Females produce testosterone (Although known as the "male" hormone, testosterone is also important to women's sexual health: it plays a key role in women's estrogen production and contributes to libido) and a lot of oestrogen, which are acid-type hormones. Each month, ovarian oestrogen is produced in large amounts, which breaks down the inner lining of the uterine wall, causing the monthly menstruation cycle. Men also produce the acidic hormones, testosterone and *Progesterone.*

These are aggressive type of hormones. They effect many different cellular changes from the breakdown of tissue to the increased growth of all types of tissue, from hair (pubic, facial, etc.) to muscle tissue. These hormones affect sexual behaviour, increase blood flow and cause erections. These acid-type hormones in men and women are naturally counterbalanced by the body with the production of progesterone and other steroids, which are anti-inflammatory and produced in the adrenal glands. When these acid-type hormones are over-produced, or not balanced by steroids, they can cause *inflammation* in tissues. This is seen as fibroids, endometriosis, hormonal imbalances and ovulatory disorders.

Okay, let us understand the basic biology behind this. The ovaries are two almond-shaped glands found in the female of a species. The ovaries have two functions. One is to produce the reproductive cell (ovum) and the other is to produce hormones. In humans, the ovaries are found on each side of the pelvic cavity, each attached to the uterus. Each ovary consists of two parts: the cortex (or outer portion) and the medulla (or inner portion). The cortex (outer portion) consists of mainly various types of follicles (small sacs). Each follicle (or sac) has an ovum (egg) and a small, yellow endocrine gland (corpus luteum). This gland (corpus luteum) secretes both oestrogen and progesterone. It should be noted that pro-hormones from the adrenal glands are necessary for proper progesterone production in the corpus luteum. The FSH (Follicle Stimulating Hormone) from the hypothalamus induces the release of the ovum (egg). The oestrogen-releasing hormone – the LH (Luteinizing Hormone) - comes from the anterior portion of the pituitary gland. **These two are vital for proper ovulation.**

Oestrogen must always be counterbalanced by a steroid called progesterone. Progesterone is a steroid produced in the ovaries and the adrenal glands. Progesterone needs a pro-hormone, DHEA, produced in the adrenal glands, to be properly produced. Therefore, when the adrenal glands are hypoactive, this can affect the production and release of progesterone, leaving a woman "oestrogen dominant". This causes a domino effect, creating extensive cellular acidosis, and leads to ovarian cysts, uterine fibroids, fibrocystic issues, female cancers and other conditions.

Menstruation is a monthly ovulation cycle where oestrogen (an acidic hormone) triggers cellular bleeding in the uterus. I call this "God's way of cleaning the house" each month. In this way, if the ovum (egg) becomes fertilized, its home will have been cleaned and prepared. It should be noted here the importance of progesterone, which is a steroid produced in the ovaries and in the adrenal glands. Adrenal progesterone (or DHEA-induced ovarian progesterone) is essential to stop the action of oestrogen and its effect upon the uterine tissue. If progesterone (an anti-inflammatory steroid) is not being properly produced because of a hypo-function of tissue, a woman will develop ovarian cysts, uterine fibroids, bleeding problems, atypical cell formation, endometriosis and cancers.

Reproduction 101

Go over this section on male and female reproduction with your partner. It's important for both of you to understand each other's reproductive system.

Contrary to what you might think, most couples do not conceive the minute they start trying. In fact, the average healthy young couple who has regular sexual intercourse has only about a 20 percent chance of conceiving each month. That's why it takes most young couples about five or six months to conceive their first child, and why it takes older couples – who have a lower chance of conceiving each month – even longer. You may think you learned everything there is to know about making babies from those late night chats with your school girlfriends or from your buddies. However, having sex at the right time of the month is *a prerequisite* for getting pregnant; and there's a lot more that must happen *at the right time and in the right manner for conception* to occur.

If you are like most of us, you learned more myth than reality – and probably more about how **not** to get pregnant than about getting pregnant. If you've forgotten what you learned in your secondary school biology class – or just didn't pay much attention – it's a good idea to review the facts about what it really takes to conceive. Conception is not a simple process but a multiple-step, multifaceted process. At any point, one or more elements may not be working up to par – or may not be functioning at all. For conception to occur, three key factors must be in place:

A *well-functioning* female reproductive system

A *well-functioning* male reproductive system

Effective sexual practices

The Female Reproductive System

The female reproductive system visualized from the lower portion of the female body consists of the following main parts: the vagina (the lowermost segment), cervix, uterus, Fallopian tubes, and ovaries (the uppermost segment). These highly specialized structures have some common features:

1. Some structures – such as the vagina and cervix – produce mucus, a substance that – depending on its consistency – can either facilitate or interfere with conception

2. Some – such as the uterus and Fallopian tubes – contract or undulate rhythmically, serving to move cells and tissues along the reproductive tract.

3. Others – such as the ovaries – release hormones at specific times during a woman's menstrual cycle, as well as produce eggs.

- **Vagina:** This lower structure of the female reproductive system is a long, tube-like vault. The vaginal membranes secrete a mucus that keeps the vaginal tissue soft and slippery, facilitating intercourse.

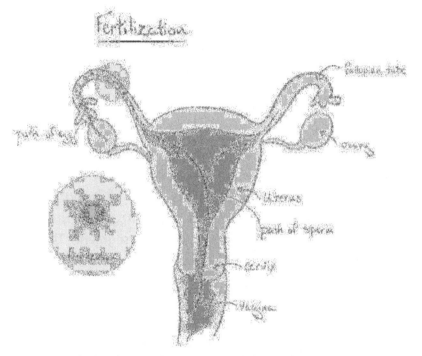

The female reproductive system after sexual intercourse.
On entering the female reproductive system, sperm follow
the direction of the arrows shown in the figure.

Picture source: www.khanacademy.org

- **Cervix:** At the end of the vagina is a small, circular area called the cervix, which leads into the uterus, or womb. The cervix has several purposes:

4. It helps protect the uterus and other reproductive organs against invasion by bacteria, fungi, and viruses.

5. During menstruation, the endometrial lining of the uterus is shed and expelled through the cervix.

6. It's through the cervix that sperm enter the uterus as they try to swim up to the Fallopian tubes.

7. During childbirth, the cervix dilates to allow the foetus to pass through its uppermost portion, the birth canal. The cervix also produces mucus, which changes consistency throughout the menstrual cycle. During most of the cycle, when a woman's not fertile, a small amount of very thick cervical mucus is present. This consistency tends to trap sperm, blocking them from entering the uterus easily. But that's okay. No eggs are yet available to be fertilized anyway. In contrast, cervical mucus becomes watery and abundant during ovulation. This helps sperm swim more easily through it and up into the uterus and Fallopian tubes, on their journey to a mature egg.

    In the fast-paced world that we live in, taking time to drink water seems like a huge task. One thing I check first when a client visits with "vaginal dryness" is water consumption level. For clients that have very busy schedules, I have them get a big calibrated drinking bottle/jug and have them set hourly reminders for water consumption – mucus is simply water-based so if you're not drinking enough water, your body will prioritize the water you're drinking for other body functions.

- **Uterus:** Located within the protection of the woman's pelvis, the uterus is thick-walled and muscular. It resembles an inverted sack. It is here that a fertilized egg normally implants itself in the uterine lining, is nourished, and matures for nine months until labour and delivery. During labour, the uterus contracts rhythmically and powerfully to move the foetus out of the womb into the birth canal and out through the dilated cervix and vagina. During menstruation, the uterus also contracts, though less violently, to expel the unfertilized egg and shed endometrial tissue.

  The position of the uterus is described by the direction in which it leans inside the pelvis. In 80% of women, the uterus leans forward – this is called an anteverted uterus. If the uterus leans forward but bends in upon itself, it is called anti-flexed. Sometimes a woman is told she has a 'tipped uterus'. This merely means that her uterus tends to tilt backward toward her spine. A tipped uterus is also known as a retroverted uterus. When it is tipped backward but bends in upon itself, it's called retroflexed. It's not unusual to have a tipped uterus, and it doesn't necessarily mean that you can't conceive, as some old wives' tales suggest. The walls of the uterus are lined with tissue called the endometrium, which responds to hormone changes throughout the menstrual cycle. It is the endometrium that sheds and sloughs off during menstruation.

- **Fallopian Tubes:** On each side of the uterus is a long, muscular structure called the Fallopian tube or oviduct, which serves as a conduit for the passage of eggs to the uterus. Each part of the Fallopian tube is lined with cells covered with microscopic hairlike projections – called cilia – that move in a wavelike manner to help guide the eggs through the tubes. The ends of the Fallopian tubes are delicate, funnel-shaped structures called fimbria that catch the eggs as they are expelled from the ovaries. The Fallopian tube lining itself produces a nutritive medium to nourish the eggs. Both the contractions of the Fallopian wall and the beating of the cilia move a fertilized egg to the uterus for implantation.

- **Ovaries:** Last but certainly not least are the all-important ovaries. These olive-sized and almond-shaped structures, found just beneath the Fallopian tubes and to each side of the uterus, contain eggs, each called an ovum. Every egg is actually housed in a bubble-like structure called a follicle. Each month, several eggs mature and normally one is released from its follicle. Most women have two ovaries, but if a woman only has one (either because of genetic or surgical defects), the other takes over the monthly menstrual cycle functions.

The Journey Towards Conception

Although only a single sperm is needed to fertilize an egg, about 300 million sperm are released with each ejaculation. Such large numbers are released to ensure that a high percentage of normally shaped, mobile sperm are able to swim fast enough up to meet with an egg as it moves down the Fallopian tube. The sperm actually travel in a relatively straight line up the vagina, through the cervix, into the uterine cavity, and finally into the Fallopian tube and hopefully into the welcoming arms of a mature ovum. This process can take anywhere from about 45 minutes to 12 hours. Sperm are actually carried through the Fallopian tubes by contraction of the tube muscles and the beating of the tubal cilia, as well as the movement of the sperm themselves. The chance of conception is diminished considerably if a man doesn't have millions of normally shaped, fast-moving sperm. The good news is that recent medical advances have helped men with low, or even very low, sperm counts to produce children. Despite this enormous, mobile army, only a few hundred or thousand sperm reach the Fallopian tube where the egg or eggs are. The other hundreds of thousands are lost.

Here are some of the problems sperm may encounter:

- Many sperm are killed by the natural vaginal environment.

- Cervical mucus may be too thick to allow the sperm to penetrate it and enter the uterus.

- Sperm movement may be so poor that too few can survive. In rare cases, the cervical mucus may contain antibodies that can incapacitate sperm. It's unclear, however, how significant these antibodies are in preventing pregnancy or causing infertility.

- Once out of the vagina, sperm movement may be

hampered by structural damage in the uterus or tubes, making it mechanically difficult for sperm to reach an egg. Of those sperm that reach the cervical canal, half enter the wrong Fallopian tube in search of an absent egg. Of those that enter the correct Fallopian tube, many are lost in the maze of the tube's folds. During this journey, the remaining sperm will undergo a process called capacitation, which gives them the capacity to penetrate and fertilize an egg.

In all these, you will agree that pregnancy is not an instantaneous event.

When everything goes right:

- The woman must ovulate a healthy, ripe, fertilisable egg.

- Fallopian tubes must be unobstructed in order to receive the egg.

- The couple must have sexual intercourse prior to or at the time of ovulation.

- The man must ejaculate millions of healthy, viable sperm deep into the woman's vagina.

- Many sperm must travel through the cervix into the uterus and finally into the open Fallopian tubes.

- The egg must be fertilized in the Fallopian tube and then travel back into the uterus.

- The fertilized egg must implant itself in a hormonally primed, normally shaped uterus, and grow into a healthy embryo.

Money Saver Tip

If you must use lubrication, look in your kitchen rather than the drug store. Egg whites and milk are good substitutes for commercial products . And they'll be easier on your pocketbook and your partner's sperm.

CHAPTER 2

||||||||||||||||||||||||||||||||||||||||||||||||||||||||||||||||||||||||||||||||||||||||

*"It is contradictory to desire to birth a child
and live a lifestyle that inhibits one"*

- Chika Samuels

||||||||||||||||||||||||||||||||||||||||||||||||||||||||||||||||||||||||||||||||||||||||

Factors Affecting Fertility

Your body is your child's first home and I often ask my clients "How baby-friendly is your child's home?", referring to your body. Choosing a healthy lifestyle is one of the best things you can do to maximise your chances of having a healthy pregnancy and baby. Your lifestyle choices must reflect your desire to bring a child into this world. Most of the following lifestyle choices apply to both women and men. However, because women are the ones who become pregnant and give birth, it's especially important that they choose a healthy lifestyle and avoid hazardous substances and behaviour.

The World Health Organization estimates that nearly 190 million people struggle with infertility worldwide and the number of couples seeking medical assistance is steadily rising. Among couples unable to conceive, infertility is partially or wholly attributable to a male factor in approximately 50% of cases. A variety of conditions can affect male reproductive potential to different extent and they often coexist. Some of these substances and behaviours are listed below:

Tobacco and Its Smoke

It's fairly well known that cigarette smoking increases the risk of spontaneous abortion and low-birth-weight babies. But did you know that smoking can increase the time to conception as well? Researchers aren't sure why, but they think that cigarette smoking reduces some types of oestrogen production and depletes egg supply. Smoking interferes with Fallopian tube motility (movement), embryo cleavage, blastocyst formation, and implantation; it has also been linked to a whole host of problems from ectopic pregnancies to miscarriages. Smoking can also cause premature menopause, thus shortening the amount of time you have to conceive. Babies born to mothers who smoke are at increased risk of being born prematurely, having low birth weight, having birth defects, and dying from Sudden Infant Death Syndrome (SIDS).

It's easy to say "but I don't smoke", but if you live in a house or work at a place where smoking is a routine affair, you are exposed to what is called "second-hand smoke". Research has shown that the chemicals in the smoke can reach the mother's blood and be passed on to her unborn child. It goes without saying that once the baby is born, it should be protected from exposure to all forms of tobacco smoke. Smoking also interferes with male fertility. It can decrease sperm production, motility, and morphology (shape). Men who smoke have sperm counts that are 15% percent lower than those of non-smokers. Indeed, a small study published in the *Journal of Fertility and Sterility* found that sperm counts rose dramatically – at least 50% and as high as 800% – in men who stopped smoking. The sperm of smokers are also more likely to be abnormal and less likely to be able to fertilise an egg. Other studies confirm that quitting smoking appears to improve the sperm of men who have low sperm counts or poor quality sperm.

Alcohol

Most people know by now that it's important to avoid alcohol during pregnancy because it can cause foetal alcohol syndrome. Drinking during pregnancy can also cause miscarriages, stillbirths, and preterm deliveries. Drinking while trying to conceive can also be risky. In fact, the Surgeon General, the U.S. Department of Agriculture, the U.S. Department of Health and Human Services, the American College of Obstetricians and Gynecologists, and the American Academy of Pediatrics all recommend that women not only abstain from drinking alcohol during pregnancy but while trying to conceive as well. Some studies have found that the chances of conceiving in any given cycle decrease with increasing alcohol consumption. One recent study in Denmark, found that moderate drinking did not affect the time it takes to conceive. Moderate drinking is defined as no more than one glass of alcohol a day for women and no more than two glasses a day for men.

A drink is typically defined as 5 ounces of wine, 12 ounces of beer, or 1.5 ounces of spirits. If you do decide to drink while trying to conceive, fertility experts recommend that you drink no more than four drinks a week. Also, only drink in the first part of your menstrual cycle before you ovulate and abstain from alcohol during the second part until you menstruate. A client once asked, *"I love a particular alcoholic brand for ladies, it is very mild and I take it right after my menses when I am sure I am not pregnant. Is that permitted on your fertility programme?"* First, no form of alcohol is permitted on the SoPrecious fertility intervention programmes, no matter how small, if you are serious about taking home a healthy baby. As a lifestyle coach, I've found that when it gets down to making the hard call of get rid of some negative lifestyles choices, people are not as ready for a change as they project.

For instance, for women who are light drinkers, most women don't know precisely when they conceive. If they do drink when trying to become pregnant, they may unknowingly be putting their pregnancies and babies at risk.

For example, I was already 6 weeks pregnant and was already entering the theatre for a surgery when they ran a random blood pregnancy test that revealed I was pregnant *(Get inspired as you get a free downloadable e-book of my story at www.soprecious.ng)*. So my stance is, why drink at all if this journey to having a newborn is that important to you? Do you know alcohol consumption increases the IVF failure rate by 2 fold? What this means that if the consensus in the IVF world is that you need 3-5 cycles to take home a healthy baby – adding alcohol to the equation may mean 6-10 IVF cycles to create your ultimate outcome.

This is the type of "numbers game" that is NOT in YOUR favour. Truth be told, you may not even need IVF if you work to remove all of the major obstacles currently standing in your way. Trust me, I have nothing against exploring other options for having a baby. I had two failed IVF cycles and still gave birth to a healthy baby after I took time to address some critical factors that were keeping me from my goal. Fertility is a "WE" sport and this applies to both partners. Alcohol can interfere with male fertility as well. Heavy drinking in men can cause a reduction in testosterone and a decrease in the volume and density of sperm. In addition, men who drink excessively often suffer from reduced libido and erectile dysfunction. If you need support to identify critical factors that may be hindering you from conceiving, our SoPrecious one-on-one intervention programme may just be for you and your partner.

Illicit Drugs
Everyone is aware that illicit drugs such as marijuana, cocaine, and so on can be dangerous to both the mother and her developing foetus. However, you may not be aware that many illicit drugs can also interfere with fertility. Marijuana, for example, can shorten a woman's menstrual cycle, thus decreasing the chances of conception. In men, marijuana and other illicit drugs can lower sperm count and impair sperm quality, upset hormonal balance, and even cause impotence. Be cautious when taking prescription or over-the-counter (OTC) medication. No OTC medication is harmless unless you have asked a certified pharmacist or your doctor. You must be careful about what you ingest (especially if they are supplements or medicine) when you are trying to conceive. Women who take birth control pills should stop taking them at least six months before trying to

conceive. It might take that long for a woman's reproductive hormones to get back to normal.

Sleep

Adequate sleep for optimal fertility is 8 hours of sleep each night and 9 hours in bed. During our intervention sessions with some intending parents, we found that a good sleep atmosphere could be a factor to consider improving for optimal conception chances. The reproduction room must *dark, quiet, clean, comfortable and conducive* for a restorative time of rest. Please give attention to each word in italics in the previous sentence.

Most homes have different forms of electronics in the bedroom. Removing electronics from the bedroom is one of the dares in the 7-Day SoPrecious Fertility Dare. I do not get it when someone says "I am trying to sleep", yet they are fiddling with their mobile phone. Bright lights have been proven to delay the onset of sleep by putting melatonin under. Melatonin sure plays a key role in egg quality and sperm production. Avoid bedside snacks as these jolt sleep homeostasis hence affecting sleep quality. This was one of the minor factors I identified when I ran this programme for myself. Lots of people underestimate the key role that adequate sleep in the right environment plays.

Replace bedside computers with hard-copy books or get a copy of your SoPrecious Lifestyle Visualizations Book. We need to teach these habits at home including teaching our children the habit of going to bed early. For example, I have screen time allocation for my son and we run a friendly structured home programme where there must be assigned time for everything including adequate rest. This is necessary for the expectant mom because important systems like the adrenal glands are rejuvenated between 11pm and 1am and if your body is awake at that time, the toxins jump right back to the liver, causing fertility and health issues.

Caffeine

A good number of urban women consume at least 100 mg of caffeine a day in the form of coffee, tea, soft drinks, or chocolate. It's what welcomes you to work and what keeps you awake at the workstation and at home. While running this programme, I noticed I was the only one that took organic herbal tea instead of coffee at the office hence I always had my own cup of organic tea so I wouldn't be tempted to indulge in coffee like everyone else. Like I often say, If you do not know *exactly WHY* you are choosing "A" over "B" and do not have the right choices for "A" available, you will most likely indulge "B".

Caffeine has been proven to inhibit ovulation, cause menstrual cycles to be irregular and causing difficulty in conception. Even when conception occurs, caffeine increases the likelihood of miscarriage as it disturbs the uterine lining which in turn prevents implantation of the fertilized egg. Women who do not consume coffee are twice as likely to become pregnant than those who moderately consume same. Caffeine decreases the number of eggs retrieved via IVF. Caffeine is not found in coffee alone. Caffeine is found in teas, soft drinks, energy drinks and chocolate, cocaine, LSD, cannabis and more.

A cup of black or green tea typically contains less caffeine than coffee.

1 can of energy drink = 80mg caffeine

1 cup of tea = 50mg caffeine

1 can of soft drink=50mg caffeine

100g bar of milk chocolate = 20mg caffeine

There is some evidence that more than 250 mg of caffeine a day increases a woman's risk of endometriosis and tubal-factor infertility. (There are approximately 300 mg of caffeine in three cups of coffee.) Women who consume more than 500 mg of caffeine take longer to conceive than women who don't, and an intake of more than 500 mg of caffeine has also been reported to increase the risk of a miscarriage. Fertility experts recommend that women who are trying to conceive limit their caffeine intake to a maximum of 250 mg a day[4]; that is, fewer than about three 8-ounce cups of coffee a day. Caffeine crosses the placenta into the foetus and has a prolonged metabolism of around a 15 hour half life. What this means is that if a mother has a 200mg caffeine at a 9am morning meeting, she will still have 100mg in her system at midnight and the body does not get rid of this till 3pm next day.

Consuming 100mg of caffeine per day *(1 small cup of coffee or 2 cups of tea)* increases the risk of having a baby with low birth weight by 7%. Low birth weight increases the risk of the child developing diseases like obesity, high blood pressure and diabetes later in life. Caffeine has not been found to have a detrimental effect on male fertility. On the contrary, there is some evidence that caffeine may increase sperm motility, thus increasing the

---

4. *https://www.ncbi.nlm.nih.gov/pmc/articles/PMC3121964/*

chance of conception. Consumption of caffeine in males increases the levels of the reproductive hormones, testosterone and sex hormone binding globulin (SHBG). This increase however damages the sperm DNA, hinders sperm production and causes a decline in all the criteria for healthy sperm (size, shape number of the sperm and its ability to move swiftly to reach an egg).

BMI and Weight

WHO estimates that 39% of adults worldwide are overweight and 13% are obese. Two of the key ingredients in disease prevention are eating a healthy diet and maintaining a healthy weight. Being either overweight or underweight can interfere with fertility. One of the best ways to determine if you are over- or underweight is by evaluating your Body Mass Index (BMI). BMI is your weight in kilograms divided by your height in meters squared (kg/m^2). If math is not your thing, don't panic!

Check out the BMI tables at *www.asrm.org/Patients/FactSheets/ weightfertility.pdf and www.consumer.gov/weightloss/bmi.htm*; they have already done the math and metric conversions for you. It is simply calculated by **weight (kg) / height (m^2)**. A BMI of 20 – 25 is associated with higher conception rates and lower miscarriage rates than those above or below this range. If you are overweight, losing a few kilos now could make a big difference to your ability to conceive. Another good measure is body fat or skinfold thickness, but it requires the use of a caliper by a health-care provider or in a gym. Body fat is measured in percentages; normal body fat is between 22% and 25% for women, and 15% to 18% percent for men. If you are overweight, lose weight! Our SoPrecious sustainable lifestyle management program has weight control is a key subject.

Extra weight in a woman can increase insulin levels, which may cause the ovaries to overproduce male hormones and stop releasing eggs. Being overweight also contributes to the development of diabetes, a risk factor for infertility. A renowned recent study (The LIFEstyle study) was the first large randomized controlled trial (RCT) to investigate the effects of a six month lifestyle intervention among obese infertile women who intended to become pregnant. Women in the intervention group had significantly more natural conceptions and a comparable rate of ongoing pregnancies. The reduced intake of sugary drinks improved insulin sensitivity, which can be explained by the association between sugar intake and insulin resistance.

The prevalence of obesity, an important cardio-metabolic risk factor, is rising in women. Lifestyle improvements are the first step in treatment of obesity, but the success depends on factors like timing and motivation. I have found that Women are especially receptive to advice about lifestyle before and during pregnancy. The pre-pregnancy period provides the perfect window of opportunity to improve cardio-metabolic health and quality of life of obese infertile women, by means of a lifestyle intervention. The study also revealed that obesity reduces fertility.

Current international guidelines state that lifestyle improvements are the cornerstone of primary prevention and treatment of obesity and cardio-metabolic diseases. Obesity is a global health problem. It impacts not only cardiovascular diseases but also on many other related health disorders. Obesity may adversely affect male reproduction by endocrinologic, thermal, genetic and sexual mechanisms. As such, obesity must be considered as a potential causal factor in male infertility; overweight and obesity were associated with an increased prevalence of azoospermia and oligozoospermia. The ASRM concluded in their *'Obesity and reproduction: a committee opinion paper committee opinion'* paper in 2015 that 'obesity in men may be associated with impaired reproductive function. [5] It is strongly recommended that males presenting for fertility evaluation should be counselled about weight-loss strategies when the BMI and waist circumference data demonstrate obesity and especially morbid obesity.[6]

The higher the weight, the greater the reduction in sperm quality. The study found that the partners of overweight men not only had a decreased chance of conception, but those who did become pregnant were at an increased risk of miscarriage. The problems were most pronounced in men with BMIs of over 30. If you're underweight, try to put on some weight, as women with BMIs under 17 kg/m^2 or whose body fat levels are 10% to 15% below normal are at increased risk of anovulatory infertility. Anorectic and bulimic women are at especially high risk of having fertility problems.

The age of onset of diabetes and pre-diabetes is declining while the age of childbearing is increasing. There is also an increase in the rate of overweight and obese women of reproductive age; thus, more women entering pregnancy have risk factors that make them vulnerable to hyperglycemia during pregnancy. Gestational diabetes mellitus is associated with a higher incidence of maternal morbidity including caesarean deliveries, shoulder

5. *A committee opinion Practice Committee of the American Society for Reproductive Medicine. Fertil Steril 2015. b;104:1116-1126*

6. *The diagnosis of male infertility: an analysis of the evidence to support the development of global WHO guidance—challenges and future research opportunities- https://www.ncbi. nlm.nih.gov/pmc/articles/PMC5850791/)*

dystocia, birth trauma, hypertensive disorders of pregnancy (including preeclampsia), and subsequent development of T2DM (type 2 diabetes mellitus). In this large European study, a modest increase in protein content and a modest reduction in the glycemic index led to an improvement in study completion and maintenance of weight loss. For a complete listing of the glycemic index of more foods, see www.glycemicindex.com

Am I Overweight?

"It is not logical that millions of modern adults and children around the world are suddenly becoming insulin resistant"

— John M. Poothullil —

Being Overweight as It Affects Males

Increased weight in males disrupts hormones, reduces testosterone production from Leydig cells in the testes and increases inflammation in the body. The number, ability to swim, size and shape of sperm is decreased by the impact of being overweight. Excess weight hinders the hormones from acting as they should – particularly Ghrelin, which stops testicular function causing poor sperm health. The heat that obese men encounter around the testes induces oxidative stress and sperm damage. This is the reason we take this factor very seriously for men that drive long distances to work or drive professionally and even more for those that operate seated powered industrial vehicles.

Eating a healthy and varied diet may be a key part of maintaining good overall health. However, there are certain vitamins and food groups that could have a greater impact on reproductive health than others. Dietary intervention is one of the key provisions of our intervention programs as we prepare a bespoke diet plan to suit the needs/ peculiarities of each client. A later chapter deals with some recipes to explore. Aspects of a male's diet may have an impact on his fertility. Consuming a diet rich in fibre, folate, and lycopene as well as consuming fruit and vegetables correlates with improved semen quality. A high amount of antioxidants has been demonstrated to increase semen quality, compared to low or moderate amounts. Antioxidants help remove the excess ROS (reactive oxygen species) in the seminal ejaculate and assist in the conversion of ROS to compounds that are less detrimental to cells. If there is more ROS than the local antioxidants can remove, it results in oxidative stress. Oxidative stress can result in sperm protein, lipid and DNA damage and sperm dysfunction. Another study reported that vitamin E and selenium decreased levels of malondialdehyde (MDA), a marker for damage done by reactive oxygen species on sperm cells & increased spermatozoa motility.[7]

Here are the key elements of achieving successful weight loss.

- Eat nutrient rich whole foods that is balanced in protein, fat and carbohydrates.

- Re-educate yourself about healthy portion sizes. Use smaller plates.

- Practice mindful eating each day – even for the first few bites of each meal.

7. *Effect of antioxidant intake on sperm chromatin stability in healthy nonsmoking men. Silver EW, Eskenazi B, Evenson DP, Block G, Young S, Wyrobek AJ, J Androl. 2005 Jul-Aug; 26(4):550-6.*

- Exercise most days of the week, getting your heart rate in the training zone for at least 30 minutes. Always get out and walk after a medium to large-sized meal. Exercise improves fertility.

- Find ways to reduce anxiety and manage stress. There is converging evidence on female body-stress response and hormones involvement. Mindfulness-based stress reduction is an excellent tool for managing stress and has proven to be helpful in managing imbalanced eating behaviours, depression and other stress related concerns.

- Use the Hunger Scale to find the place of satisfaction vs absolute fullness.

Eating Disorders.

A review of diet and lifestyle is where we want to start from. Underweight people are encouraged to eat every hour (the 100 calories every hour diet). If you can't manage that, eat six times consistently every day. Drinking healthy caloric fluids is another good way to support weight gain, as long as it doesn't interfere with food eaten at meals. The term "eating disorder" sounds medical so many think it must be an illness that is far from them. Today's urban people consume mostly street-food, road-side snacks and quick meals all day long and most of these are made up of endocrine-distrupting and sperm-quality damaging ingredients.

Consumption of these kind of foods project 'eating disorder' as a frequent critical factor that some of clients have had to face head-on and address. Eating disorders such as anorexia and bulimia are associated with fertility problems and negative attitudes to pregnancy, according to a UK study. The research also revealed high rates of unplanned pregnancies in women with a history of anorexia, suggesting they may be underestimating their chances of conceiving. *Professor Philip Steer, Editor-in-chief of BJOG: An International Journal of Obstetrics and Gynaecology* said:

> "Eating disorders have important clinical consequences, especially in women. This research shows that more women with eating disorders are unprepared for pregnancy and will therefore require more support during the antenatal and postnatal period."

Eating disorders are known to cause disruption to a woman's menstrual cycle, with substantial weight loss leading to hormonal changes that might prevent ovulation.

Being Overweight as it Affects Females

Some recent studies have revealed that weighing too much can interrupt normal menstrual cycles and throw off ovulation or stop it altogether. There is a wide range of body shapes and sizes that can be healthy and the number on the scale is not that relevant as a measure of health. Body Mass Index (BMI) and waist circumference are two measurements that, when used together, can better help to assess for a healthy weight. The Body Mass Index (BMI) Chart is the same for males and females. It is simple to use. First, find your height on the chart and then find your weight on the chart. The number where they cross is your body mass index (BMI).

Achieving a Healthy Weight

Weight balance, through attention to a balanced diet, portion control, daily exercise and mindful eating is key. Weight balance for optimal fertility includes a healthy body mass index (BMI) between 20 and 25 and a waist circumference (WC) of less than 35 inches for women and less than 40 inches for men. A healthy BMI of 20 to 24 is considered the *"fertility zone"*. Women with a BMI less than 20 may be at an increased risk of infertility. I had a client that was too lean; coaching her to organically but steadily gain between 2.3 or 4.6 kg was enough to restart ovulation and menstrual periods. Women with a BMI above 25 may be at an increased risk for metabolic syndrome, type 2 diabetes and polycystic ovary disease. Being overweight also reduces the chances that in vitro fertilization or other reproductive technologies will succeed while increasing the risk of miscarriage, high blood pressure (pre-eclampsia), gestational diabetes and the chance of needing a caesarean section.

I had a client whose key critical identified factor was being overweight, in just two weeks into our bespoke SoPrecious fertility intervention program, she steadily lost 7% of her initial weight and this immediately set her ovulation in order. Ideally losing 5-10% of overweight has been proven to improve ovulation. This number alone isn't the whole picture. I have had intending mothers with high muscle mass who appeared to have a higher BMI. However, when used along with waist circumference measurements, it does give a more comprehensive picture of their weight status. Waist circumference is a measure of the health risk associated with too much stomach fat. Men with a waist circumference more than 102 cm (40 inches) and women with a waist circumference more than 88 cm (35 inches) are at increased risk of developing weight related health problems.

To measure your waist circumference, place the tape measure half way between your hip bone and your lowest rib. This will be about 5 cm (2 inches) above your belly button. Wrap the tape measure around you in a circle. Make sure the tape measure is level all the way around. The tape measure should not push in or indent the skin. Relax, exhale and measure.

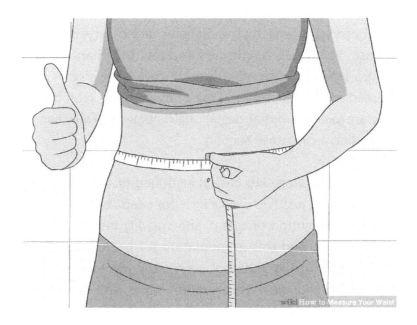

A small change in weight can make a difference. Even a change of 10% has been found to have a positive effect on health. You can increase your chances of getting pregnant by achieving and maintaining a healthy weight. The National Infertility Association reports that 30% of infertility cases are due to weight extremes, which can alter hormone levels and throw ovulation off schedule. On the other hand, women who are underweight, with a body mass index below 18.5 *(18.5 to 24.9 is considered normal)*, may experience irregular menstrual cycles or stop ovulating altogether, according to the American Society of Reproductive Medicine. Those who regularly participate in high-intensity exercise — such as gymnastics or dancing, have an eating disorder or follow restricted diets — often are at an increased risk.

Excess weight increases risk of miscarriage, stillbirth, while excess weight in women with PCOS (Polycystic ovarian syndrome is the leading cause of infertility among woman of childbearing age) disrupts ovulation and conception opportunities. Obesity increases the risk of gestational diabetes (a condition that 14% of pregnant women all over the world are faced with), this condition increases preterm risk and Caesarean delivery and invariably birthing a large-for-gestational age baby and this in turn increases the child's risk of obesity, heart disease and blood sugar issues.

Avoid going on fad diets, as these can deplete your body of nutrients it needs for pregnancy – this is why I do not recommend vegan diets or similar diets as well as popular weight loss programmes for those on a fertility journey. Being vegetarian or being on a vegan diet is actually terrible for your fertility. There have been lots of studies that show that most vegetarians and vegans do not get enough amino acids and essential and non-essential amino acids to make good quality sex cells, like egg and sperm. Women who have too much stored energy often have difficulty conceiving for other reasons, many of which affect ovulation. Stored energy includes insensitivity to the hormone insulin, an excess of male sex hormones and overproduction of leptin, a hormone that helps the body keep tabs on body fat. There are many reasons why weight can get out of balance over time. Some people are too sedentary and some eat an unbalanced diet. Some are unaware of portion sizes. Others are emotional eaters. The solution to weight problems will depend on **why** the weight is out of balance. It is very seldom a simple issue of balancing calories in with calories out. Identifying these WHYs and agreeing on the HOWs is the bridge that our fertility intervention sessions creates for intending parents struggling with weight.

Mindful Eating

We do food every single day! Conscious Eating is a big step toward Conscious Living. Quality and Quantity of Food is directly related to our Health and state of mind. We can use food to help us recover from Stress and Disease. Not taking food seriously will eventually lead to Stress or/and Disease."

— Natasa Pantovic Nuit —

Mindful eating is a way to approach the daily ritual of eating with more awareness. If practised regularly, it can transform our eating and our health. With each day, and each meal, we have an opportunity to slow down and **notice what** we are eating and **how it feels** in our body. Slowing down, noticing, paying attention makes it easier to connect with ourselves and our body. This is important level of personal awareness to cultivate at any time, but mindful eating offers valuable benefits during the preconception period. Studies show that mindfulness practices are very effective in reducing stress, anxiety, depression and unbalanced eating.

Mindful eating can focus our attention and calm our mind. It is deceptively simple and, at the same time, very, very difficult. It is difficult because we live in a fast-paced culture with many distractions that keep us from ourselves. To slow down can seem excruciating at first, but it is worth persevering. We invite you to try mindful eating – start with just one meal or even for the first few bites each time you eat. Mindful eating as a way of eating can help you slow down and tune in to your body, mind and spirit. It offers a daily way to practice mindfulness (paying attention, on purpose, in the present moment, without judgment), which has been shown to be helpful to manage stress, blood sugar, blood pressure, anxiety, depression and imbalanced or disordered eating.

Hunger Satisfaction Scale – A Tool to Manage Consumption

Evidence currently suggests that chewing may decrease self-reported hunger and food intake, possibly through alterations in gut hormone responses related to satiety.[8] Stress is an inseparable part of our lives, and most of us deal with it quite efficiently, without major health problems. This

---

8. *Effects of chewing on appetite, food intake and gut hormones: A systematic review and meta-analysis. (https://www.ncbi.nlm.nih.gov/pubmed/26188140)*

means young and otherwise healthy women may experience only temporary and probably reversible effects of stress on their reproductive function. "But for women already suffering from fertility problems, even a minor impact on their ovarian function may influence the chance and timing of conception." There could be a relationship between eating, stress and reproductive function. "Because ghrelin is so closely linked to hunger and feeding, these findings very broadly suggest that our eating habits may be able to modify the effects of stress on fertility.[9]

The 'Hunger Hormone' and Reproductive Health

Ghrelin is a metabolic hormone that triggers feelings of hunger, increases food intake and promotes fat storage. It's also released when we are stressed; ghrelin is part of the reason we want to eat when we feel emotional or under pressure. Neuroscientists at RMIT have been exploring the role of ghrelin in healthy reproductive function, and implications for fertility. In this new pre-clinical animal study, they investigated how ghrelin may mediate the effects of chronic stress on the ovarian primordial follicle reserve.

Female mammals are born with a fixed number of these "immature" follicles, which do not regenerate or regrow if they are damaged. While the majority of primordial follicles will die and never complete their development, a small proportion will eventually develop further to become preovulatory follicles. This means the fewer "immature" ones you have, the fewer "mature" follicles later in life that can release an egg cell for

---

9. *Dr Luba Sominsky Associate and Professor Sarah Spencer published in the Journal of Endocrinology*

fertilisation. The study found that female mice exposed to chronic stress had significantly fewer primordial follicles. But when the researchers blocked the effect of ghrelin on its receptor, they found the number of primordial follicles was normal – despite the exposure to stress.

"The length of the female reproductive lifespan is strongly linked to the number of primordial follicles in the ovary," Sominsky said. "Losing some of those primordial follicles early on is often predictive of earlier reproductive decline and deterioration. This research is in early stages, with many steps to go before we can translate this clinically. But getting a better understanding of the role of ghrelin in all of this brings us an important step closer to developing interventions that can keep these critical parts of the reproductive system healthy."

Hunger is a completely natural sensation and not something to be feared. The Hunger Scale we have created for you to use is a way to describe your level of hunger and help you to recognise when the best times to start and stop eating occur during your day.

Level E: The stomach is uncomfortably empty and is a deviation from the self-referral path of comfort – try to eat before getting to this level.

Level 0 – 1: As digestion takes place, there is no remnant of food in your stomach from the previous meal – your stomach seems empty and you feel hunger. You are not starving but there is a definite need to eat.

Level 2 – 4: This range describes how you feel as you

are comfortably continuing to eat and food is being comfortably digested. There is no sensation of hunger.

Level 5: You start to feel satisfied.

Level 6: You are full, but at the point of maximum comfort.

Levels 7 and 8: Your stomach is completely and uncomfortably full.

Level F: You can't eat another bite and the thought of food makes you sick.

Introduction to the Mindful Eating Practice

1. When you sit down at the table, take a deep breath and relax. Check in with your feelings. Notice and observe them.

2. Clear away any distractions such as the television, computer, phone, books, and newspapers.

3. Notice the food on your plate. Notice the temperature, aroma, colour and arrangement on the plate.

4. Appreciate the food, the farmers and all the work involved in bringing this nourishment to you. Find a place of gratitude.

5. Start eating slowly. Take one bite of food, put down your fork and chew your food thoughtfully. Become aware of the flavour, pleasure and health that the food is giving you.

6. Listen to your body. Notice when you are satisfied or

when foods don't agree with you. Continue to breathe. Continue to eat and just notice. Notice when you feel satisfied. Notice when you feel full. Ask yourself; What am I really hungry for? How hungry am I? How much do I need to satisfy that hunger? How do I feel when I eat that food? What am I feeling right now? Let the feelings flow through and just keep noticing them.

7. Continue eating your meal, resisting the pull to rush through or distract yourself.

8. When you are finished eating, pause and take a deep breath. Appreciate yourself for taking care of yourself. The secret to mindful eating is the daily practice. i invite you to try eating mindfully each day. Start with the first few bites of each meal and then try a mindful meal each day, until it becomes part of your rhythm. Mindfulness practices have been shown to be very effective in helping people manage emotional and imbalanced eating problems, as well as depression and illnesses associated with stress.

Being Underweight

Women's health practitioners have known for ages that body fat and energy stores affect reproduction. Women who don't have enough stored energy to sustain a pregnancy often have trouble ovulating or stop menstruating altogether. Changing weight is a challenge whether you are trying to lose or gain weight. However, the body needs some body fat for hormonal balance. One of the questions we ask at our fertility sessions with our intending mothers are why a person is underweight. Some of the reasons could be:

Stress: The Fertility Killer

Stress is defined as an inability to respond appropriately to the environment. The resulting physical response can manifest as a myriad of nervous system complaints including insomnia, restlessness, nervousness, or a general state of agitation. In some cases, the immune system becomes compromised, resulting in everything from an increased susceptibility to colds and flu to hormonal imbalances and chronic disease states. Stress puts the body into a "fight or flight" mode, which increases the cortisol hormones and neurochemicals and selectively redirects the blood flow to the brain, the eyes, and the musculoskeletal system. This adaptive mechanism allows us to escape from danger. However, most of the stressors we experience in twenty-first- century life do not require the "fight or flight" response, yet our bodies haven't adapted as our environment has changed. Our stress response may be triggered by an endless number of situations: overwork, environmental pollution, emotional factors, worry, and so on. Far too many of us live with high stress levels most of the time. Unfortunately, the stress response preferentially redistributes blood flow away from the gastrointestinal, endocrine, and reproductive systems, all of which are non-essential to the "fight or flight" response.

In October 2001, an important study of the effects of stress on conception was published. Doctors at the University of California, San Diego, examined the success rates of a group of women undergoing gamete intrafallopian transfer (GIFT) or IVF (two forms of ART). The study concluded that women with the highest rated life stress levels were 93% less likely to become pregnant and achieve a live birth than women who scored lower on the stress scale. Day in and day out, our bodies still need to eat, relax, and reproduce, but under stress, these systems won't get the blood flow they need to function efficiently. Blood quits flowing to the stomach, hence we get ulcers and have a wide range of digestive complaints.

Blood over-nourishes certain parts of the endocrine system and starves others, so we don't produce the right balance of hormones needed for a healthy menstrual cycle. And the poor uterus and ovaries are ignored altogether! In addition, the hormone adrenaline, which is released by the adrenal glands during conditions of stress, inhibits the utilization of progesterone, one of the key hormones of reproduction. How do we handle stress while dealing with the hustle and bustle of city-life? Most people are not aware of how much stress their bodies are subjected to until it breaks down with an illness to get their attention.

First, step away from any guilt you may feel about how you have been living up to this point. Begin by relaxing. Believe your journey has been perfect (even with all of its shortcomings) up to this point. Resolve to make whatever changes you can to support greater health for your mind, body, and spirit. The greatest gift you can give your future child is to love, honour, and accept yourself. The decline of male fertility, particularly associated with advancing age, poor lifestyle choices and environmental factors play an important role on natality, and its consequences on the future on human population makes this an important public health issue in this century. Thus, modification of lifestyle through a structured programme of educational, environmental, nutritional, physical exercise and psychological support, combined with the use of nutraceutical antioxidants can prevent infertility and therefore, may help couples to obtain better quality of life and improved possibility to conceive spontaneously or optimize their chances of conception.[10]

Age

Age has adverse effects on fertility in both sexes, but more so in women. The optimal time for a woman to conceive is from her mid to late 20s. However, many women in their 20s may not be married, they may be busy pursuing their education or careers, or they just may not yet feel ready to start their families. What I will share below on how age affects fertility are all facts but these many times have been defied by couples whose faith & commitment to lifestyle modifications has brought their desired children to earth. Fertility in women starts declining significantly after age 30, and even more rapidly after 35. A woman under 30 has about a 20% chance of conceiving each month. By the time she reaches 40, her chances of conceiving drop to only 5 percent each month. Approximately one in three women aged 35 or older will have a fertility problem. By age 40, two out of three women will be infertile. Older women are also significantly more likely to have miscarriages, as well as babies with birth defects.

Why is this? After age 30, hormone levels start declining and egg production starts to deteriorate. At birth, a female has as many eggs as she will ever have in her lifetime – over a

---

10. *Lifestyle and fertility: the influence of stress and quality of life on male fertility. Department of Movement, Human and Health Sciences, Section of Health Sciences, University of Rome "Foro Italico", Rome, Italy. https://www.ncbi.nlm.nih.gov/pubmed/30474562*

million. By the time a girl reaches puberty, she has about 300,000 left, and only 300 of those will ever be ovulated. The older a woman is, the older her eggs, and older eggs are not as fertilisable as young eggs. Because they've been around for a lifetime, they've had decades of exposure to various adverse elements – viruses, X-rays, drugs, and environmental toxins. As a result, older eggs are much more likely to carry chromosomal abnormalities that can cause such disorders as Down syndrome. In addition, older women may not be in as good physical health as younger women. The older you are, the greater the chance that you've had a serious illness – such as an STD, diabetes, thyroid disease, or hypertension – that can interfere with fertility and your ability to carry a child to full term. . This explains why I often say that fertility is a lifestyle as lifestyle choices should be resounded and upheld in our schools and young adult groups even before they are grown to want to breed children.

Fertility in men also decreases with age, although not as dramatically as for women. Starting at about age 25, sperm cell production starts decreasing, and the sperm that are produced tend to have decreased mobility, thus hindering their ability to reach and fertilize an egg. Men over the age of 35 are twice as likely as men under 25 to take more than a year to impregnate their partners. One reason may be that older couples tend to have sex less often than younger couples. As men grow older, they tend to have lower levels of testosterone. This, in turn, affects their sexual drive as well as their ability to achieve and maintain an erection, which, of course, can affect their ability to impregnate their partners.

Older men are also more likely to have medical conditions, such as atherosclerosis (hardening of the arteries) or diabetes, which can impair sexual ability. Ageing can cause genetic mutations in the sperm cells, potentially leading to genetic defects in their offspring as well as miscarriages. Indeed, pregnant women who are 35 or older with male partners over the age of 40 have a significantly increased risk of miscarriages. Regardless of the age of the father, if conception does occur, the age of the mother has serious implications for the outcome of a pregnancy. Not only does the chance of conceiving decrease the older one gets, the chance of miscarriage increases as well. This may be due to the various medical conditions such as those mentioned earlier, or to genetic problems in the embryo. Older women are also at increased risk of having stillborn babies, low-birth-weight babies, premature deliveries, and Caesarian sections. As a result, their babies are at increased risk for serious health problems. Babies of older women are also at risk for having genetic or congenital problems. BUT if you're older, don't despair. The good news is that the majority of older women who do carry a pregnancy to full term and give birth to healthy babies. This is one of the needs that this book fulfils; to not just help you get pregnant but support you in conception attempts and through birthing a healthy baby.

Money Saver Tip

Make your own meals as opposed eating out. A little bit of proactiveness makes it easier. Plan your meals ahead and shop deliberately. It is cheaper and at least you are sure that you are feeding your body and baby the right nutrients to foster conception. Engage at our blogs to get all the tips for reading labels and intentional nutritional shopping.

CHAPTER 3

||||||||||||||||||||||||||||||||||||||||||||||||||||||||||||||||||||||||||||||

*"He that wants to embrace must
proceed with open arms"*

- Chika Samuels

||||||||||||||||||||||||||||||||||||||||||||||||||||||||||||||||||||||||||||||

Lifestyle Choices Necessary for Fertility Improvement

A lifestyle choice is a personal and conscious decision to perform a behaviour that may increase or decrease the risk of injury or disease. Despite an understanding of what constitutes a healthy lifestyle, many people lack the behavioural skills to CHOOSE everyday to sustain these good habits. Nevertheless, healthy lifestyle modifications are possible with appropriate interventions just like ours. Lifestyle factors can be modified to enhance overall well-being and they are ultimately under one's own control. They play a key role in determining reproductive health and can positively or negatively influence fertility.[11] A healthy lifestyle is known to be of importance for women, especially when they are planning to get pregnant, since negative lifestyle factors may contribute to impaired reproduction and a lower chance of having a healthy child. Such negative factors include smoking, drinking alcohol and over-use of other drugs, being underweight or overweight, unhealthy dieting, harmful infections, exposure to environmental hazards, and an adverse medical history.

If you are ready to take charge and do what it takes to turn your dream of parenthood into reality, then this book with enormous tips for lifestyle and fertility interventions is for you! Lifestyle factors are behaviours and circumstances that are, or were once, modifiable and can be a contributing factor to sub fertility. Fertility is the capacity to produce offspring, whereas fecundity is a woman's biological ability to reproduce based on the monthly probability of conception. Clinical infertility is defined as the inability to become pregnant after 12 months of unprotected intercourse. The causes of infertility are wide ranging including diagnoses such as, ovulatory disorders, tubal disease, endometriosis, chromosomal abnormalities, sperm factors and unexplained infertility. The relationship of lifestyle factors such as diet, physical activity, smoking, and alcohol intake, to chronic diseases is well known. There is good evidence that diet, lifestyle and nutritional supplementation can impact fertility. Infertility can be caused by a huge number of factors: hormone

---

11. *Lifestyle factors and reproductive health: taking control of your fertility.*
    https://www.ncbi.nlm.nih.gov/pmc/articles/PMC3717046/

imbalance, polycystic ovarian syndrome, endometriosis, anovulatory cycles, physical blockage, inadequate hormone production, short luteal phase, lack of lutenizing hormone, high levels or prolactin, and many others.[12] Below are some lifestyle choices that are recommended for women who are considering child bearing:

1. Exercise

You can always bet on the good endorphins that exercise rewards. Beyond weight loss, I love the reward that the body releases after some sort of intentional work-out. It's a cascade of feel-good hormones (endorphins). These endorphins are Mother Nature's antidepressants, lowering your stress level and boosting your sense of well-being. Exercise burns calories and helps regulate your insulin levels, reversing some of the metabolic imbalances that are contributing to weight gain and fertility issues. Just walking for 30 minutes every day has a positive effect. Any exercise at all is better than no exercise. Always move your lymphatic system. Everyone has a stagnant lymphatic system to one degree or another. All your cells need to eat and excrete, and your lymph system is your sewer system. Your lymph nodes are your septic tanks. Keep them cleaned out!

For the urban woman, there may never be time to exercise so you need to make a deliberate effort to incorporate more activity into your daily routine. For example, parking your car a distance from your destination, taking stairs instead

---

12. *https://www.ncbi.nlm.nih.gov/pmc/articles/PMC4345758/*
    Indian journal of medical research, Association of western diet & lifestyle with decreased fertility

of an elevator, hiring a trainer, registering in a gym enroute work, taking early morning/ evening brisk walks with your partner, etc. Everyone knows that being physically fit is good for you. Exercise and maintaining a healthy weight go hand in hand. As we've seen, being overweight can hinder your chance of conceiving, and exercise is one of the best ways to keep weight down. I had a client who insisted that she has her weight under control and does not need exercise- she said she does not eat much and controls hungry and has an hour-glass figure to show for it but is too busy for exercise. When we looked at the critical factors affecting her frequent miscarriages- lack of exercise and healthy meals were major critical factors we identified, so my question for her was "How important is this birth journey to you? Are you willing to adjust your schedule to address these critical factors?"

For optimal fertility, I do not advise getting caught up with this new wave of "get slim fast", "keep slim regimes without exercise" all over social media. Simple exercises (like walking or swimming) are extremely important in moving your lymph system, especially in your lower extremities. Deliberately allow yourself sweat especially if your daily lifestyle does not involve much physical activity. Your skin is your largest eliminative organ. Keep it clean and stimulated with skin brushing, hot-and-cold showers, and by sweating. While exercise in itself won't help you conceive, it will keep your heart healthy and your blood pressure down, both of which are important for a healthy pregnancy. On the other hand, too much exercise can interfere with fertility. For example, female athletes and women who engage in very vigorous sports or activities such as marathon running are predisposed to menstrual irregularities and may have trouble conceiving.

2. Supplementation

The food we eat does not give us all the nutrients that our body needs for optimal fertility hence the need for supplementation. I often get the question, *"What supplements must I take to enhance my fertility?"* It Is not all known brands that are effective for the purpose of use and when we have a closer look at their fertility profile and then the active ingredients of the supplements that they are using, we discover that they have been using those ignorantly and they are a false representation of the adequate supplementation that their body really need for optimal fertility. Firstly, a prescription for supplements should be focused on organ health optimization. Supplementation is a session we take very seriously in SoPrecious fertility interventions and there is no "one size fits all" approach for this as every intending parent has varying critical factors that varying supplementation, different active ingredients and varying dosages will address.

For Supplementation, Buying over the counter self-prescribtions will be doing yourself a great disservice. You will do yourself a huge favour by using "practioner-prescribed only products". What is shared here are options you could run by your practioner before use or engage us for more detailed assessment and review to be sure that what you are getting are the building blocks that your body needs for optimizing your fertility.

Generally, DHA (Docosahexaenoic acid) is an essential fat for egg development and helps to optimise egg quality. If you have been taking high EPA: DHA, no harm done – but for optimum male and female fertility, I have found a high DHA:EPA ratio to be the best. The higher the DHA, the more a supplement will cost. Visit our site www.soprecious.ng for recommended brands with the highest DHA ratios. For optimal fertility, you want a much higher ratio of DHA to EPA (at least 2:1) for optimal fertility. I do not recommend any over-the-counter vitamins and minerals for several reasons including poor quality, insufficient strength, wrong dosage for individual requirements. Taking appropriate vitamins and supplements like Folic Acid – one of the B vitamins – is not only important for the health of the mother, it is essential to the health of the developing fetus. Folic Acid contributes to the neural tube development in early pregnancy and inadequate amounts can lead to serious neurological and spinal birth defects. It's recommended, therefore, that women of childbearing age have a minimum of 400 micrograms (.4mg) of folic acid daily. Although many foods contain folic acid – such as whole wheat grains, brown rice, fortified cereals, oranges, spinach, and beans – it's often difficult to get an adequate amount through diet alone.

To be safe, it's recommended that all women who are planning to conceive start talking folic acid supplements three months before they even start trying to conceive and for at least the first three months of pregnancy. Other essential vitamins and minerals include iron and vitamin A. But make certain you do not take more than 5,000 units of vitamin A each day. Men should also consider taking vitamin supplements, especially zinc. Between 15 and 30 mg is considered safe for both men and women; anything above that amount can be dangerous. Take a calcium supplement if you aren't able to manage getting 1000 mg/day from your diet. Choose calcium citrate with added magnesium and vitamin D. However, if you eat a whole food, mostly plant-based diet, you should be able to absorb enough calcium from your diet. The foundation supplements that nearly all couples need include a high quality multivitamin, fish oil, which has a high DHA: EPA ratio and coenzyme-Q10. Those supplements are going to build the basic foundations of what you need so buy the best quality that you can afford. For women and men really on this fertility journey, coenzyme-Q10 is extremely important for women. You're looking at least 600mg per day, and for men, you're looking at about 300mg to 400mg, but again the quality of this really makes a huge difference.

High quality food is always the best source of nutrients. Supplements can be useful in fine-tuning a healthy diet and providing extra support for fertility. Supplementation is based on you as an individual, on your diet, lifestyle, and health goals. The Nurses' Health Study found that women who took a multivitamin or mineral supplement at least six days a week had a higher fertility rate. Prenatal multivitamin mineral supplements are generally recommended for women trying to conceive. They contain 0.4 to 1.0mg of folic acid and B vitamin that is involved in central nervous system development of the early foetus. A high iron intake of at least 40mg/day is associated with increased fertility. The current recommended daily intake (RDI) for iron is 13gm/day for women of childbearing age. Most prenatal supplements contain iron, but they also contain calcium. It is important to note that a combination of both inhibits the absorption of the other, so I usually recommend an iron-free prenatal taken in conjunction with, but not at the same time of day as, an additional liquid iron supplement. Lean meat (simply meat with low-fat content eg skinless chicken, turkey and red meat are iron-rich foods and delivers a form of iron that is easily absorbed by your body)

Selenium is a trace mineral that protects cells from oxidative damage. It is also needed for iodine metabolism and a healthy thyroid. Selenium is found widely in plant foods, depending on the quality of the soil. Brazil nuts, eggs and oatmeal are some of the best sources of selenium in the diet. The recommended daily intake is 55mcg/day. Selenium is often found as part of an antioxidant formula. B12 (cobalamin) supplementation is strongly recommended for people following a vegan diet. B12 is available through Brewer's Yeast, which can be sprinkled on food, or through a supplement of 2.6mcg/day or 200mcg/day. Recent research links Vitamin D to cancer prevention and a supplement of 1000IU/day is recommended for all adults. A question I am often asked is, "With so many OTC drugs, how can one get a quality fertility supplement?" A good quality supplement is well balanced, highly absorbable and free of contaminants or artificial ingredients. Vitamin D – 1000 IU/day is what is recommended.

The best supplements available to date are organic food-based supplements. They are highly absorbable and include a probiotic supplement that enhances absorption and digestibility. Most of them have an excellent prenatal multivitamin/mineral supplement for women and a one-a-day capsule without iron for men.

Note: Supplements for men should not contain extra iron because studies have shown a link between supplemental iron intake and heart disease in men.

As one of the many B vitamins pregnant women should take, a folic acid supplement may increase your chances of conceiving twins. While the reasons are still unclear, Professor of Clinical Sciences Bength Källén of the Tornblad Institute in Lund believes that "it is possible that folic acid somehow increases the probability of multiple ovulation or implantation of more than one egg." When it comes to creating a daily intake regiment, the National Institutes of Health recommends adult women consume 400 micrograms, pregnant women consume 600 micrograms and lactating women consume 500 micrograms.

Avocado, Ugu *(fluted pumpkin leaves)* bitter leaves, water leaves, Efo shoko, African egg plant leaves, African basil leaves, spinach, broccoli, kiwis, carrots, sweet potatoes and asparagus are all good sources of folic acid. You may take twice the amount of recommended dosage of folic in pregnancy if you are trying to conceive twins. If you would like to increase your chances of conceiving twins, take a daily 400mg to 1000mg of folate supplement and consume Vitamin B9-rich foods (these include green leafy vegetables, beets, lettuce, citrus fruits). Taking more than the suggested amount of folic acid is not known to cause any harm to the body, as the excess is removed in the urine.

I must state here that most valuable ingredients of vegetables are killed during preparation. Most forms of vegetable soup preparations in Nigeria for instance involves prolonged cooking and this leaves the consumer with just nice-tasting bare soup and not a vitamin-rich vegetable sauce. I share in a chapter, simple ways to include vegetables, seeds and nuts in your daily consumption and also how to make a wholesome vegetable soup or sauce.

To get a bespoke supplementation & fertile meal plan for your peculiar situation today, contact us to book a session with our fertility expert.

Money Saver Tip

*If you are at beginner stage with exercise
and you are on a budget; do not invest yet
in a gym place registration. Start with early
morning brisk walks or runs with your partner
and find online and practice various mild
workouts that you can do in your room or
at your office desk. The key is consistency.*

||||||||||||||||||||||||||||||||||||||||||||||||||||||||||||||||||||||||||||

CHAPTER 4

"Your Body is your licence to earth;
understand & treat it with respect"

- Chika Samuels

||||||||||||||||||||||||||||||||||||||||||||||||||||||||||||||||||||||||||||

Body Awareness

The sense of ownership of one's body is important for survival, e.g., in defending the body against a threat. However, in addition to affecting behaviour, it also affects perception of the world.[13] Let us take a closer look at ovulation; I call it "A Woman's Key to Conception". Pinpointing ovulation can further ensure that you have sex at the right time. Unfortunately, the precise time of ovulation is typically only known retroactively; that is, after it's already occurred. Pregnancy is unlikely to occur even a day after ovulation. The trick, then, is to anticipate when ovulation is most likely to happen. Luckily, there are some easy, fairly accurate,

---

13. *https://www.ncbi.nlm.nih.gov/pubmed/28826500*

non-invasive ways of determining when your ovulation is. One real key to correct ovulation period recognition is by body monitoring.

Monitoring your body

Certain body signals can indicate impending ovulation and even ovulation itself. One such sign is called *mittleschmertz*, a feeling that many women experience in their abdominal region around the time of ovulation. Some feel a twinge, some a sharp pain, and others mild discomfort in or around the ovaries. One of the best signs of ovulation, however, and one most women experience, is a change in the quality and quantity of the cervical mucus during the menstrual cycle. By checking your cervical mucus, you can tell whether you're approaching ovulation. A few days before you think you may ovulate, insert a CLEAN finger into your vagina and get a small sample of mucus from around your cervix. Then try to stretch the mucus between your finger and thumb. If the mucus is thick, pasty, sticky, and/or opaque, you're unlikely to conceive because sperm can't live or swim in this hostile environment. But if the mucus is clear, thin, and stretchable, it's an indication that you're approaching ovulation. You're most fertile when you can stretch the mucus an inch or more without it breaking – a characteristic of cervical mucus called *spinnbarkheit.* Your partner's sperm will also be able survive and swim more easily to your awaiting egg in this friendly, moist environment. The reason women can become pregnant for up to six days before ovulation is because sperm can survive in this "non-hostile" cervical mucus for several days.

Please note that lack of cervical mucus and having thick cervical mucus are not always signs that you aren't ovulating. Some women produce good cervical mucus at the time of ovulation, but it stays in the cervical canal, making it difficult to detect. And, infection or prior cervical surgery can have adverse effects on cervical mucus, causing it to thicken. But for most women, the changes in cervical mucus are very reliable predictors of ovulation.

Charting your Temperature

Another way to find out if and when you ovulate is by keeping a basal body temperature (BBT) chart. This usually involves tracking your temperature each morning. The BBT is sometimes used to determine the LH surge which is an indication of ovulation. To chart your BBT, you should take your temperature orally, rectally, or with an ear probe every morning before getting out of bed, or if you prefer, later on in the day as long as it's the same time each day. You should then plot the temperature changes on a chart, and mark which days you menstruate and have sexual intercourse.

Over two or three months, the typical chart of an ovulating woman will show a pattern of a slight temperature rise (0.4 to 1.0 degrees F) at mid-cycle. The rise in temperature remains fairly level until about the time of menstruation, at which point the temperature drops. This is called a *biphasic pattern* and is a good indication that you ovulated. If no temperature elevation is apparent for several months – what's called *a monophasic pattern* – you're probably not ovulating and should see a reproductive endocrinologist as soon as possible. Some couples mistakenly think that they should have sex when they see the temperature rise. Although the LH surge usually occurs a day or two before ovulation, by the time the temperature rise is apparent, you've probably already ovulated. If so, it's too late to conceive. Indeed, there have been no documented cases of a pregnancy occurring the day after ovulation

Unfortunately, BBT cannot determine ovulation ahead of time, only after the fact. For that reason, many doctors don't recommend its use. However, it can give you some indication of your ovulation patterns before seeing a doctor. It can also help you and your doctor determine whether your cycles are abnormally long or short. Another advantage is that it can be an indirect indication of an early pregnancy. If an egg does become fertilized, your temperature will probably continue to stay elevated instead of dropping as it does when you're about to get your period.

Use of Ovulation Kits

Body basal temperatures are great. Ovulation kits are not so great. They're often inaccurate and don't enable you to gain an understanding of your cycle on the same level as charting your BBT allows. If you don't know your cycle, ovulation kits are not going to be enough. Make sure you start charting your cycles to know exactly what your body does. This will enable you to figure out the lengths of your follicular and luteal phases, for example. With this type of insight about your cycle, you become able to find answers that are actually going to help you.

Menstrual Phases & Fertility Window

The menstrual cycle is commonly characterized with respect

to specific milestones and events denoting various phases. The first day of the ovarian cycle is defined by the onset of blood flow (menses), which also marks the beginning of the follicular phase.[14] Ovulation occurs approximately halfway through the menstrual cycle, denoting the onset of the luteal phase. These two phases are often further subdivided into early-, mid-, and late-follicular, as well as early-, mid-, and late-luteal as characterized by levels of estradiol and progesterone. Specifically, progesterone is very low throughout the follicular phase, whereas estradiol is very low during the early follicular phase and is followed by a rise, as the follicle develops, that peaks sharply in the late follicular phase. The end of the follicular phase is concomitant with a surge in luteinizing hormone (LH), which is caused by the increase in estradiol. The LH surge heralds ovulation and the formation of the corpus luteum, which secretes progesterone, marking the start of the luteal phase. Approximately half-way through the luteal phase (mid-luteal), progesterone peaks and estradiol has a secondary peak.

Table 1

Characterization of Menstrual Phases

		Follicular			Ovulation		Luteal	
	Menses	Early	Mid	Late		Early	Mid	Late
Days based on 28-day cycle	1–4	4–5	5–7	8–12	13–15	16–20	21–23	24–28
Progesterone								
Absolute Values (ng/mL)	< 2	< 2	< 2	< 2	2–20	2–20	2–30	2–20
Relative Change	Stable	Stable	Stable	Mild Increase	Increase	Large Increase	Peak	Large Decline
Estradiol								
Absolute Values (ng/mL)	20–60	20–160	100–200	>200	>200	100–200	100–200	20–60
Relative Change	Stable	Mild Increase	Large Increase	Primary Peak	Large Decline	Mild Increase	Secondary Peak	Moderate Decline
Luteinizing Hormone								
Absolute Values (mU/S/mL)	5–25	5–25	5–25	5–25	25–100	5–25	5–25	5–25
Relative Change	Stable	Stable	Stable	Stable	Peak	Stable	Stable	Stable

(Figure 1; Table 1)

14. *(Yen et al., 1999)*

Research recommend that a menstrual cycle may be considered "normal" as long as a menses occurs every 23–32 days, with the follicular and luteal phases lasting anywhere from 10–20 days and 9–17 days, respectively.[15] Variation in menstrual-cycle length depends on when the follicle begins to develop (producing predominantly estradiol) and the viability of the corpus luteum (which produces the peak of progesterone). This cycle variation is subject to a variety of both genetic and environmental factors.[16]

- **Follicular Phase:**

This is the first pre-menstrual phase. For most likelihood of fertility, this should not be than 10 days else the egg quality can be compromised.

- **Luteal Phase:**

This is the second half of your menstrual cycle after ovulation (the phase before ovulation is called the follicular phase). The number of days for each phase is a critical factor in failure or victory of conception. For example, a 10 day luteal phase constitutes an infertile cycle, even if conception occurs. A victorious luteal phase must be a minimum of 12 days and ideally 14 days.

It takes 10 to 12 days for implantation so if it dropped at eight DPO (days past ovulation (DPO), your luteal phase was too short for implantation. The luteal phase ends when your progesterone drops. A basal

---

15. *(Cole et al., 2009)*

16. *(https://www.ncbi.nlm.nih.gov/pmc/articles/PMC4821777/#R58; Determining Menstrual Phase in Human Biobehavioral Research: A Review with Recommendations.*

body temperature of 36.3C and above is ideal in the follicular (1st half) phase and 36.5C and above in the literal (2nd half) of cycle. The SoPrecious Conception Cycle Demystified programme was created for this purpose. When it comes to sex and getting pregnant, your window of opportunity is relatively small and seemingly harmless additives like the wrong types of lubricants can really knock back your chances of success. When a woman begins her mid-cycle peak of ovulation, I recommend trying to conceive every second day and once a day is perfectly fine. But you really want to be guided by mucus changes, and by what your basal body temperatures are telling you retrospectively. These are the things that are going to be most important.

Generally speaking, mucus will peak 1 to 2 days prior to ovulation occurring, so if you know that that's the case and if you know your particular pattern, when that mucus peaks, you know, "Okay, now this is the time to start trying to conceive." Now, some fertility illnesses like PCOS for example, can be tricky because the body can go through several attempts of ovulation and you generally will get a lot of stretchy mucus at different times of the month, which can be a little bit confusing. Then you're not so sure whether you have ovulated unless you're charting your temperatures. Even the predictive kits can be a bit off from time to time. Depending on where you are in your cycle, they won't necessarily work. As a result, I find the easiest and most effective way of pinpointing ovulation and actually being able to figure out what's going on is

BODY AWARENESS

a combination of fertile signs, charting, and basal body temperature charting. Yes, I know, it is a slow process and may take a couple of months for you to get the hang of it. Yes, it can be a little bit off. Some days, you probably just need to confirm whether you have ovulated or not. To do so, I would just check my temperature for a couple of days in a row and just figure it out and then I wouldn't need to chart any more.

That truly is something that is very useful once you actually get the hang of it, provided that you look at it from the perspective of "I'm gathering information about my body, I want to know as best as I can what it is that I can do in order to optimize it", then that's the best way to approach it so it doesn't seem like a chore. Set a reminder to do this at same time of the day and insert at the same spot every day. As far as frequency and regularity of sex, you should aim for at least every second day. You don't want to leave it any longer than every second day. You can certainly have intercourse everyday if you wish to. It's not necessarily going to give you a better outcome and certainly twice a day is not going to give you a better outcome either. Every second day is just fine.

The one thing that you want to really make sure of is that that your partner doesn't pull out his penis too quickly after ejaculation. You want the penis to be flaccid before it's pulled out of the vaginal cavity because otherwise, it can create a vacuum that sucks out all of the sperm. In addition, it's always ideal for the female orgasm to happen around the same time or just after the male orgasm. Time of day to

99

have it? – whenever you feel like it, really. To learn how to improve your chances of conception, register today for the next The SoPrecious Conception Cycle Demystified, a three-week programme, available to couples all over the world as a fully personalized, online program and personally delivered by fertility & lifestyle specialists.

MALE FERTILITY

In an Oxford England journal published in December 2016, an article "Men's knowledge of their own fertility: a population-based survey examining the awareness of factors that are associated with male infertility" posited that male factors, such as low sperm count and abnormal sperm morphology, are primary or contributing causes in almost half of the diagnosed cases of infertility. Men were less knowledgeable about how daily activities and excessive heat sources, such as the use of laptops and frequent hot tub use, can impact male fertility. These findings highlight the importance of educating men about such health risks in order to address modifiable risk factors through health promotion activities, such as diet, exercise and stress reduction techniques. The survey proved that the more information that individuals have about fertility, the more likely they are to exhibit positive health-seeking behaviours to improve their own fertility.

The health of a man's sperm dictates three of the following very important things.

1. The ability to conceive. It is a 50-50 equation, after all.

2. Chances of a miscarriage. Scientific evidence is

now talking about the role and responsibility that oxidation of sperm or damaged sperm plays in miscarriages and pregnancy losses.

3. Ability to create that healthiest possible baby. Your baby's health is a reflection of its parents' health prior to conception.

So, it's really important to note that getting pregnant is a team effort, a couple working together to optimise the chances of conception and of course, carrying a healthy pregnancy to term. Someone once asked "Can sperm be incompatible with the egg?" Absolutely yes, it can be. Female sperm antibodies, an incompatibility with the egg for whatever reason, could reduce the sperm's exposure to the egg.

In terms of incompatibility, it's generally not the egg that is going to be affected. It is mostly the cervical mucus. Even though the egg can have antibodies to your sperm, it is usually female mucus that will kill the sperm. The result of this hostility is that the sperm never is able to get to the egg. The best way to prevent that is by wearing condoms anytime you have sex other than the times that you're actually trying to conceive. This will reduce the female immunological response to the sperm, if there is one there. When trying to have a baby, timing conception and intercourse are also going to be vital. Miscarriages are a 50:50 equation when it comes to egg and sperm quality – there are 7 category reasons for miscarriages. Get more details on our blogs at www.soprecious.ng

Sperm: The Key to Male Fertility

Just as the ovulation of a viable egg is the key to female fertility, ejaculation of healthy sperm is the key to male fertility. You might hear that it takes only one egg and one sperm to achieve a pregnancy, but that's only partially true. While it does take one egg, millions of sperm are required to ensure that one sperm will be healthy and strong enough to fertilize that one egg. There are approximately 100 to 300 million sperm in the average ejaculate; if there are fewer than 200 million sperm, the chances of conception are diminished. Every man produces many sperm that are malformed (poor morphology) or are incapable of travelling fast enough in a straight line (poor motility) to make the trip up to the uterus and finally the Fallopian tubes. The cervical mucus filters out most of the abnormal sperm. Many thousands of healthy sperm now need to make the long trip – a process that can take anywhere from 5minutes to 24hours. When the remaining healthy sperm meet up with the egg in the Fallopian tube, they bombard the egg's protective coating, called the cumulus.

Thousands of sperm die in the process. It takes about an hour for the egg to be stripped of its cumulus, at which time new sperm arrive and try to penetrate the egg's next protective membrane, *the zona pellucida*. Only those sperm that have been capacitated can penetrate the membrane and fertilize the egg. One – and, it is hoped, only one – will succeed. If more than one sperm penetrates an egg, called polyspermia, fertilization is unlikely to occur. But if it does, the woman will undoubtedly not even know she had conceived because she's likely to have a very early miscarriage. From this complex process of survival of the fittest, you can see why it's necessary for a man to have an adequate number of sperm per ejaculation, and why the majority of those sperm must have good morphology and motility.

These three key factors – *sperm count, morphology*, and *motility* – can be evaluated easily by semen analysis. You see why I emphasised the need to see a doctor in an earlier chapter. Most male fertility issues start getting better with similar dietary adjustments. I found that most of these issues are rooted in lifestyle choices like addictions to caffeine, alcohol, dairy and trans fat. The male partner needs to avoid environmental oestrogens and dietary sources of free radicals including saturated fats, hydrogenated oils, and trans fatty acids. Stop or reduce all unnecessary medications, especially antihypertensives, antineoplastics, and anti-inflammatory drugs, which can impair sperm production. It's important to increase consumption of legumes and soy (which is high in phytoestrogens and phytosterols), and include vitamins C, E, and B12, beta-carotene, folic acid, and zinc, and herbs such as ginseng, which increase production of testosterone and helps with sperm production. Supplement your diet with the amino acids L-arginine and L-carnitine, which are especially associated with enhancing sperm production. This regimen will improve not only the quality of sperm but overall health too.

Low sperm count, low motility and low morphology are the easiest thing to fix with the SoPrecious one-on-one coaching session. Remember that new sperm are produced every 120 days so with committed changes, improvements are very likely. Here are my suggestions for improving high-viscosity sperm:

- Do the *#SoPrecious7dayFertilitydare* and adopt the lifestyle learnt.

- Book a one-on-one session with our fertility specialist because essentially what happens is that viscosity of sperm improves and decreases by decreasing inflammation, decreasing toxicity, and ensuring that the host of the sperm, is as healthy as possible.

- Avoid junk food. Make sure that your male partner is eating and living clean. Small changes, once implemented will improve high viscosity sperm.

Money Saver Tip

Invest in a digital thermometer, which is not breakable and gives a more accurate reading than a glass thermometer. Check our blogs for our recommendation of advanced ovulation calendar and fertility trackers that help you track, analyse, understand and learn the peculiarities of your own phases

‖‖‖

CHAPTER 5

"Patience is the calm acceptance that
things can happen in a different order
than the one you have in mind."

-David G. Allen

‖‖‖

Let's Talk About Sex

Timing as it Affects Fertility

There's one fairly simple – not to mention pleasurable – thing you can do to help ensure that your chances are maximized each month: Have sex often enough to ensure that you don't miss your most fertile days. So many expectant women have a false awareness of their fertile window hence miss to have sex when they should and have it when they necessarily need not. The key role of timing as it affects fertility is core of what is addressed at our intervention procedures.

Recent research has found that the average woman is fertile for six days a month – the five days before ovulation and the day she ovulates. The two days before ovulation are usually the days a woman is most likely to conceive. It's difficult to predict those two optimal days. So, to take advantage of the six-day "window of fertility," it's a good idea to "schedule" sex every other day around the time you think you might ovulate. That means usually starting on day 10 of the ideal 28-day menstrual cycle. This pattern helps ensure that enough sperm are present whenever the woman ovulates, since sperm usually are viable for 48 hours. Of course, you might prefer to cover all your bases and have intercourse every day starting around day 10. It's ultimately up to you and your partner to decide how often to have sex as long as you have it during your fertile period. There is, however, some evidence that having sex several times a day or frequent masturbation can deplete the sperm pool. In fact, the concern about depleting a man's sperm supply is behind the fairly common advice that men should save up their sperm by abstaining from sex for several days prior to their partner's fertile period.

Sperm takes a day or longer to get to the egg and the life span of an egg is a couple of days. The theory on gender is the female trait sperm do not swim as fast but have longer endurance. If you want a girl you should have sex a few days before ovulation. Male trait sperm swim faster with a lower endurance. If you want a boy, you should have sex on ovulation or the day after. My recommendation is that every second day is okay. More sex means less sperm each time for same output over all. This means that frequent ejaculations helps to reduce DNA fragmentation which is good, but having sex every second day around ovulation is enough.

Sex and Sex Drive

Sex drive is simply the desire to have sex. Women's sexual desires naturally fluctuate over the years. Highs and lows commonly coincide with the beginning or end of a relationship or with major life changes. Some medications used for mood disorders also can cause low sex drive in women. If your lack of interest in sex continues or returns and causes personal distress, you may have a condition called hypoactive sexual desire disorder (HSDD). I often advise that you don't have to meet this medical definition to seek help. If you're bothered by a low sex drive or decreased sex drive, we recommend bespoke lifestyle changes and sexual techniques that may put you in the mood more often.

"Sexual desire in women is extremely sensitive to environment and context," says Edward O. Laumann, PhD. He is a professor of sociology at the University of Chicago and lead author of a major survey of sexual practices, The Social Organization of Sexuality: Sexual Practices in the United States.Lifestyle interventions are the first step in the treatment of obesity and have shown to improve several domains of physical health, mental health and increase quality of life. A six-month lifestyle intervention in women with obesity and infertility led to more frequent intercourse, better vaginal lubrication and overall sexual function 5 years after the intervention. (Trial Registration: NTR1530, A lifestyle intervention improves sexual function of women with obesity and infertility: A 5 year follow-up of a RCT).

Research findings indicate that women with eating disorders experience more difficulties in the sexual and relationship domain. One previous study and a couple of interactions with few of our clients has found that women with eating disorders view their marital relationship as less satisfying than their spouses view it, but that satisfaction improved significantly as the eating disorder symptoms were addressed. Sexual intimacy is a fundamental aspect of healthy relationships that can be disrupted by an eating disorder, and should be assessed routinely along with other more commonly evaluated realms of functioning (e.g., social, occupational, exercise, nutritional). For lack of sex drive, I recommend that you book a one-on-one session with us for a tailored intervention to improve hormonal balance and eating disorders for sure, but anything that will wake the body is useful as a kick start. Also keep in mind that women typically truly get aroused around ovulation but still you may need intervention. Getting enough sleep, reducing stress and anxiety will be quite essential, otherwise you will be using up your reproductive hormones to make stress hormones and this is not ideal for fertility.

There's a big difference between actually having the desire to have sex but having trouble physiologically and just not being in the mood or being turned on by your partner. I often suggest you get your hormones checked first. If the results turn out okay, then you have to address what's going on. Perhaps your partner needs to work on turning you on. Find out what turns you on by yourself first and show him. What I have also experienced working with some couples is that one partner assumes the other partner should know what works for him or her in bed. We all have different love languages and for most women, sex starts before the bedroom.

Getting ready for love-making is intentional and efforts must be deliberate to achieve a desired result. Also, we look at previous personal experiences, for example, was your libido an issue before or is this a new development? The reality is that in order to be able to conceive, you really don't need to have that much sex. ***You just need to pinpoint it correctly***. There are also some things you shouldn't do when having sex. If possible, don't use vaginal lubricants. If you do prefer to use lubricants, don't use any that contain spermicides – as their name implies, they kill sperm! In addition to reading the label, it's a good idea to ask your doctor about their contents. Even lubricants without spermicides can hamper sperm motility. Body oils and creams can trap sperm, too. If you must use a lubricant, choose only water-soluble ones. Like I will always say, Of course, the best lubricant is the natural secretions of the vagina. Check our website for popular lubricants that you find in pharmacies which are actually toxic to sperm cells and also find our recommendation of safe options you can use instead.

Money Saver Tip

If you must use lubrication, look in your kitchen rather than the drug store. Egg whites and milk are good substitutes for commercial products and they'll be easier on your pocketbook and your partner's sperm.

||||||||||||||||||||||||||||||||||||||||||||||||||||||||||||||||||||||||||||

CHAPTER 6

*"Call it a clan, call it a network, call it a
tribe, call it a family. Whatever you call
it, whoever you are, you need one."*

- Jane Temple Howard

||||||||||||||||||||||||||||||||||||||||||||||||||||||||||||||||||||||||||||

Nurture of a Community – *Building Healthy Relationships*

Malcolm Gladwell tells a fascinating story in his book *The Outliers*. He describes a small town called Rosetta in the US where immigrants from a village in Italy had settled. The town is renowned for the health and longevity of its inhabitants. Residents of Rosetta are astonishingly immune to the normal North American diseases like heart disease and cancer. Researchers were at a loss to explain this phenomena as they could find nothing different in the diet or genetics of Rosseta compared to other towns in the region. Finally, they identified the differentiating factor – the community itself.

Three generations of families often lived together. Everyone knew their neighbours and people felt safe and supported. Whenever a family or individual was in difficulty, neighbours rallied together to take care of them. The researcher finally concluded that it was this culture of caring for one other that was the source of the remarkable health of the residents. More and more studies are showing that feeling connected is a potent elixir of health – lowering your blood pressure, boosting your immune system and creating feelings of happiness and well-being which are essential to making babies. Humans are social beings, and studies have shown that having a supportive community of family and friends is the most important determinant of mental and physical health.

I can't exhaustively explain to you what the benefits are, of surroundings yourself with the right kind of energy. It's important that you are in the right kind of community that inspires and rekindles the right kind of passions, feelings that are geared towards achieving your set goals. Who you have got in your space matters! Let's zoom in on YOUR relationship with your spouse. Fertility is a team affair. This is one time that both intending parents must be on same page for a common goal. I totally understand and can relate to the strain that trying for a child builds on marital relationships – I have been there but I have also noticed that the strain is not as much when the couple are "a team against the world" and refuse to allow unhealthy third party interferences.

I have discovered in practice that a lot of the time, the woman is the one that has all the facts and details and asks the most questions, Often times, men are not engaged and involved in the fertility journey to optimize their chances. Even clinical interventions like IVF focus more on what the woman must do through out the 30-day cycle. The couples need to engage on same level to optimize their fertility potential. I have met some women who are eagerly willing to go all the way with the fertility programme but are not in talking terms with their husbands or have to deal with one fight after another at home. I understand the strain that trying to conceive for years drags in the home but this is where team work comes to play. Partners need to manage each other's shortcomings, judge less, believe more, encourage more and love more.

My husband and I would often go back to our vision board when strain tried to set in and remind ourselves, "We are in this together. We are pushing for the same thing and not against each other." Most of time, a communication gap is the real issue. I find often that men disconnect because they are not educated enough to the level to make informed decisions on lifestyle choices. A lot of times, they demand answers to the questions 'Why' and 'How' and relevant responses will enable them go all in to create a great team for the family. The challenge is that when men ask these questions, women tend to feel unsupported or defensive meanwhile they are simply asking to be able to make more informed decisions and know what their roles are.A solid and robust family environment begins even before a baby enters the picture, it all begins with a solid tribe or village. If you are courageously embarking on the path of solo reproduction, undoubtedly you will have people in your life that mean a lot to you, to whom you can apply this learning. For everyone else whether in a marriage, union, whatever the way you are building your family, your relationship matters. Have fun in the process. Your relationship is critical to your fertility success and it needs to be a priority.

One of the greatest relationship quotes I have read, by relationship researcher Dr John Gottman says: "Happy couples understand that helping each other realise their dreams is one of the goals of marriage". And I couldn't agree more. Trust me, this fertility journey can make or break relationships. With this in mind, the SoPrecious fertility dare has days to focus on effective exercises for relationship building. Applying yourself to these exercises helps to discover ways and means to make it work, for you both (Get more information on our website and social media handles) The focus should be on the process not the partner and sometimes communicating needs is a minefield. It's worth the effort to reconnect, and the journey is much easier when both partners at least feel valued and understood.

Here's an exercise for you:

On a piece of paper each for you and your partner, identify your top 3 shortcomings & top 3 values. What this exercise will do is help you be aware of your spouse's needs and expectations and help your spouse be aware of yours. After taking time to identify your emotional needs, it's important that you validate your spouse's feelings and most importantly, commit to re-evaluating and meeting each other's needs as a couple. Yours may be different from his, as men and women are different, but it's still important for you both to agree.

When my husband and I did ours, my values were and still are:

- God *(faith)*

- Family *(spending time with family and creating memories)*

- Being a helper, adding value

Interestingly, his values are not so far off from mine. Ensure that this fertility journey does not turn into a "child hunt" or an obsession. Remember, don't let it take over your lives; you had a life before the baby quest, and you will have one after the baby arrives. Build a fulfilling career by focusing on personal and career development. Don't be deceived into thinking that a baby will suddenly make you joyful. Find joy now in the little things of life. Count your blessings. Get a free copy of our SoPrecious Vision board journal when you book a session with us: this fantastic tool helps you do a daily input of gratitude, supernatural childbirth affirmations, vision board for your expectations etc. With this journal, you can redirect energy and focus and make your moments of self reflection to be productive.

Self-Care

*"You can not pour from an empty
cup-Put self on your agenda"*

— Chika Samuels —

You cannot be positive or give positive energy to others if your own basket isn't full and you are feeling depleted. Women are generally so busy catering to household chores, work, business, relatives and so many other responsibilities that we do not take time to nurture ourselves. When you draw up your to-do list, remember to put yourself as priority. Some of the self-care activities you can do are reading an inspiring book, pamper yourself with SoPrecious fertility oils in a bubble bath with candles and music, or take a walk around your neighbourhood. Take time each day to meditate and connect to what's important to you and what you are grateful for.

Mindfulness

Why is infertility viewed as a life crisis? Infertility reaches into the most important areas of our lives: our relationships, our careers, our finances, and especially our sense of self. When a couple tries for a child for more than one year, worry and fear sets in, it strains their relationship as they begin to play blame games, misunderstandings grow between the couple, it affects even sibling and in-law relationships, it distracts from career and purpose pursuits, finances are at risk because money goes in the direction of everyone's opinion about what works and when all these fail, the self esteem is battered.

Infertility is typically experienced as one of the most difficult situations a couple can ever encounter. Unlike previous endeavours, efforts to conceive do not equate with success, thus attempts to gain control over a situation that lies outside one's control, only heightens a sense of insecurity. And, because infertility challenges the inherent assumption that we can have children whenever we choose – that procreation is a birthright – the inability to father a child or become pregnant becomes a personal catastrophe.

Though infertility is a medical condition, it is experienced as a redefinition of self, challenging our core identity of what it means to be a man or woman. In the process, the very qualities most needed are least accessible. Here rests a core paradox: How has it come to be, that in this very quest to bring new life into the world, we bring with us so little life of our own? Mindfulness becomes the perfect antidote for the paradoxical land mines infertility presents. It all starts from the perspective that you are whole and complete already, regardless of flaws or imperfections. Ours is based on the concept of original goodness: your essential nature is good and pure. Proceeding from this vantage point gives you freedom from the bondage of inadequacy and insecurity. The SoPrecious Mindfulness techniques are offered at our intervention sessions and these help to open the mind up to the present moment just like it is, whether it's pleasant or unpleasant, without clinging to it or pushing it away.

In our fertility intervention sessions, You learn to relinquish control not by trying to change, get rid of, or judge the situation – in this case, infertility – but rather by changing your relationship to what's happening. We provide you the vehicle to become the change itself. As you do this, you cultivate the cornerstone quality of acceptance: a state of open receptivity, a willingness to turn toward that which you resist. Paradoxically, when you accept things as they are, you are better able to assess the situation, find your strength, make wise choices, and take wholesome actions.

There is so much in life you can't control, and your efforts to try to change what you don't want only intensifies the problem. When you let go of control, insecurity, and rigidity, you open up, release, and let things be. You are shifting from the coping mechanism of control – trying to change what is – to acceptance by being with what is. SoPrecious mindfulness techniques teach you to relax, release, and let go: to breathe through every contradiction of clinging to what you want or pushing away what you don't want and to open to the unfolding process of life. Through repeated practice, you learn resistance is how you get stuck and acceptance is how you break free. More than a stress-reduction technique, SoPrecious mindfulness techniques are a way of being – a method of meeting what Taoists call "the ten thousand joys and the ten thousand sorrows" inherent in the human experience. Mindfulness cultivates the qualities you most need, such as non-judgment, patience, and trust, and transforms the most insurmountable obstacles and plights into challenges and opportunities for growth. Mindfulness challenges assumptions about who you are and why you are doing what you are doing. Through mindful inquiries, we help you look deeply into such questions as:

1. "Is infertility the obstacle, or is fertility the challenge?"

2. "Is infertility happening to me or for me?"

3. "Is my true longing pregnancy or parenthood?

4. "Is infertility the loss of a dream or a dream not awakened?"

It's not about following the prescription that leads from point A to point B; rather, it's answering the invitation to drop into your heart – to come full circle on the wheel of paradox that starts with loving yourself just as you are and ends with loving yourself just as you are. Through this gateway, you give birth to yourself.

Money Saver Tip

Be intentional in choosing those in your circle. Nurturing healthy valuable relationships take time and loads of patience and understanding but the dividends and profit is enormous and for a long time. If one falls, the other can help his friend get up. But how tragic it is for the one who is [all] alone when he falls. There is no one to help him get up.

CHAPTER 7

||||||||||||||||||||||||||||||||||||||||||||||||||||||||||||||||||||||||||||

*"Let food be your medicine and
medicine be your food."*

-Hippocrates

||||||||||||||||||||||||||||||||||||||||||||||||||||||||||||||||||||||||||||

Nutrition & Fertility

A study on protein intake and ovulatory infertility by Chavarro
JE1, Rich-Edwards JW, Rosner BA, Willett WC, Department of
Nutrition, Harvard School of Public Health, Boston, USA, reveals
that replacing animal sources of protein with vegetable sources
of protein may reduce ovulatory infertility risk. Do not miss the
point—the issue here is not meat consumption but the amino
acid building blocks for optimum egg and sperm quality—it
just that these are easiest to get from meat or animal proteins.
However, I have had a couple of clients who choose to continue
being vegetarian and I do not have a problem with that as long
as we refer for a proper biochemical, amino acid profiling of their
body *(as we always will in those cases)* and supplement with a
bespoke amino acid formulation.

These things can be done. The key is that it needs to be done properly. Furthermore, if one chooses to be vegetarian, I will suggest they really should be the best and healthiest vegetarian there ever was and there have been plenty of great traditional books dedicated to that discussion. The key here is a varied, fresh (not always half-cooked or steamed) vegetable (not carb loaded grains) diet that excludes soy of any type. Most health experts' recommendations and government-sponsored dietary guidelines agree that a healthy diet for those with child-bearing intentions should include an abundance of certain nutrient-rich foods, fruits and vegetables. These foods should contain a variety of essential nutrients as well as other compounds that are associated with lower disease risk such as fibre and bioactive substances.

A landmark study based on the Harvard Nurses Study, makes startling connections between diet and conception. This comprehensive research on diet and fertility associates a slow carb, whole food, mostly plant-based diet with a six-fold increase in fertility. Contemporary research and ancient practices both demonstrate that healthy eating for fertility is based on a **natural, whole foods, plant based, anti-inflammatory diet** that includes the following:

- Whole/ Plant Based Foods

- Slow Carbs

- Whole grains foods

- Plant protein

Whole/ Plant-Based Foods

Whole foods are minimally processed and refined as little as possible before being eaten. Whole foods provide maximum nutrients, fibre, enzymes, antioxidants and taste without added artificial flavours, colours, preservatives, sweeteners or trans fats. Whole foods are simple, local, unrefined foods, where processing is limited to enhancing digestibility (soaking, fermenting) or to food preservation such as canning, smoking, curing and drying.

Plant-based foods include a rainbow of high fibre, high antioxidant fruits and vegetables, legumes, nuts, seeds and whole grains. A plant-based diet means that most (but not necessarily all) of the diet is based on plant foods and is associated with health promotion, disease prevention and longevity around the world. I am an advocate of sourcing proteins from plants (beans, peas, lentils, nuts, seeds) and less from animals (meat, poultry, eggs, and dairy). Contrary to old ways of thinking about protein quality, plant proteins are actually an excellent source of high fibre protein.

Slow Carbs

Foods and drinks provide fuel for our body in the form of carbohydrates, fat, protein and alcohol. Carbohydrates are the body's preferred fuel source. The glycaemic index (GI) is a way to classify foods and drinks according to how quickly they raise the glucose level of the blood. It has replaced classifying carbohydrates as either 'simple' or 'complex'. There are different types of carbohydrate and the type you eat has a significant influence on fertility. Diets high in refined sugar and easily digested carbohydrates increased the odds of *ovulatory infertility*. Carbohydrates are the primary determinant of blood sugar and insulin levels. Fats and protein are digested slowly and do not have much impact on blood sugar by themselves. When blood sugar and insulin levels rise too high, they disrupt ovulation.

In fact, the study found that the amount of carbohydrates in the diet was just as important as the type. Women whose diet contained at least 60% of its calories from slow carbohydrates tended to be a healthier weight than women who generally avoided carbs altogether. There are two basic types of carbohydrates:

- Fast carbohydrates (high GI foods) bring a quick influx of glucose into the blood stream which then leads to a rapid rise in insulin. This is often associated with a quick energy high followed by a depressing low. Fast carbs include foods made with white flour, refined sugar, alcohol, candies, cookies, fast/junk food or pastries, chips, frizzy drinks or soda. Junk food is food that is high in calories but low in nutritional content while soda is carbonated water, originally made with sodium bicarbonate, drunk alone or mixed with alcoholic drinks or fruit juice)

- Slow carbohydrates (low GI foods, diets that are

rich in high fibre) are associated with improved fertility. Slow carbohydrates are a group of carbohydrates that are slowly digested causing a slower and lower rise in blood sugar after being eaten. Low GI foods include whole grains like your local brown rice, legumes, beans, and vegetables. This lines up nicely with work showing that a diet rich in these slow carbs and fibre before pregnancy helps prevent gestational diabetes- an increasingly common problem for pregnant women and their babies. Eating slow carbs help to minimize insulin resistance, regulate blood sugar, improve fertility and prevent gestational diabetes. Slow carb eaters tended to have an overall healthier lifestyle including more exercise, less alcohol and coffee, less fat and animal protein and more plant protein.

Whole Grains

Whole grains are plant foods that include all parts of the grain kernel: the bran, germ and endosperm. Whole grains contain the most nutrients including B vitamins, magnesium, chromium and fibre. They take longer to cook but are worth it for their flavour, texture and nutrition. These are the best source of complex 'slow' carbohydrates as they are high in fibre, enzymes, antioxidants, vitamins and minerals. Eat a few servings of whole grains every day, depending on your energy requirements. Refined grains are whole grains that have been processed to remove part of the bran, germ or endosperm. The more a whole grain is refined during processing, the more nutrients are lost e.g. refined" whole wheat flour, couscous, etc. These can be eaten occasionally, however should be avoided by women with PCOS or women trying to lose weight. Processed grains have been totally refined or processed to the point where there is very little nutrition left. Examples are white rice and white flour.

Some refined grains have had nutrients added back to them after processing such as enriched white bread. However, you should avoid these foods while you are following the SoPrecious Fertility Diet. Studies say PCOS patients should restrict the amount of flour products they eat, and in my view, eliminate it totally. Sprouted wheat or grains are a better choice as even whole wheat flour is processed and quickly digested and can cause rapid increase in blood sugar. To slow down the rate of absorption for flour-based foods, you can combine them with healthy fats (like almond or peanut butter- you can blend yours at home) or protein. True whole grains are: barley, large oats, brown rice, amaranth, quinoa, millet, wheat berries, spelt berries and kamut berries.

Remember – the most important element of the SoPrecious Fertility Diet is to eat WHOLE foods. Because the national food regulatory bodies ensures the manufacturers declare the ingredients of their products, one sure way you know you are eating a whole food produce is that it does not have a list of ingredients!

Plant Protein

Nuts and Seeds

Nuts and seeds are a great source of quick concentrated protein and good fats. Limit your daily intake to no more than one ounce (about 20 nuts) and choose natural organic products. For variety, try almond butter, cashew butter, and hazelnut butter in addition to natural peanut butter. Toss a tablespoon of ground flax seed on your oatmeal each morning. Try pumpkin seed butter, sunflower seed butter or hemp seed butter on your toast instead of butter or margarine.

High Antioxidant Foods

High antioxidant fruits, vegetables, herbs and spices help to decrease oxidative stress and cellular inflammation associated with decreased fertility. Organic produce has been shown to be higher in antioxidants. The SoPrecious Elixir drink offers a fantastic combination of high antioxidants; not only does it kick-start your liver's metabolism which fixes hormonal imbalances, you see the results on your skin! Let's talk about this good girl- turmeric. Turmeric is a fantastic liver tonic and like all liver tonics, it helps with oestrogen conjugation and excretion thus making it a PERFECT herb to consume in any case of hormonal imbalances especially oestrogen dominant conditions. This makes it an ideal food and herb for women with endometriosis, fibroids and other reproductive conditions.

It requires pepper to utilize the curcumin (its active ingredient), as such, it's excellent for your pepper soup, stews. I still add raw turmeric to my nut milk drinks and morning ginger loose tea. Below are two of my recipes whose ingredients are very high in anti-oxidant properties and helped address my critical issues like inflammation, fibroids and weight control.

Below is my good night ritual:

SoPrecious Golden Nut Milk Drink

Tiger *nuts (or tigernuts) are tiny tubers that grow underground. They have a sweet and nutty flavour and renowned for their milk-ability. Making this recipe takes a few simple steps. If you can't easily source tigernuts, feel free to substitute almonds in this recipe. If you use fresh tigernuts, there is no need to pre-soak them. Dried dates can be used as sugar-free way to sweeten the milk.*

Every ingredient listed below is intentionally chosen to improve libido and increase conception chances and is safe to be taken by male and female and at all phases of the menstrual cycle.

- *1 cup almonds or 2 cups of tigernut (soaked overnight, The longer they soak, the softer they will be and the easier they will be to blend into silky, smooth milk)*

- *5 dates (to sweeten)*

- *½ fresh coconut (to increase creaminess)*

- *2 Knobs of Ginger*

- *2 Knobs of turmeric*

- *4 cups filtered frozen water (plus extra water for blending)*

- *Cinnamon for spice*

(makes approx. 750ml)

Directions

If using dried tigernuts or almonds, rinse and soak in a generous amount of water overnight.

Drain soaked nuts and pour into a blender. Add in the ice cubes and a little at a time for blending, add all other ingredients. Blend on high until smooth and creamy. This usually takes around three minutes

Place a sieve bag (same type used for pap) or fine sieve, nut bag, cheese cloth over a large bowl and pour the blended mix/pulp to separate the milk from the tiger nut pulp.

A lot of people will stop here but I will blend out all the goodness from the pulp before discarding so place the tiger nut pulp back in the blender and add another 1-2 cups of water. Blend again for a couple minutes and the strain again.

This can be repeated up to three times. You can combine the milk with the first batch, or keep your batches separate. The second and third batch won't be as creamy as the first.

Once you've finished, pour the milk into a glass jar and store in the fridge for 3-4 days.

Nut milk has tendency to coagulate in the fridge, simply shake before each use. You will also notice that the frozen water helped the "butter" from the nuts to coagulate at the base of your blender, gently scoop this out for your organic face masks/ body butter.

Below is my good morning elixir:

SoPrecious Organic Herbal tea
To help build sustainable lifestyle habit of water consumption, I often advise that my clients carry along jar of drinking bottle or drinking cup (at least half a litre).

This will serve as a reminder to refill to drink water and also ensures you have clean filtered water before and when you need it instead of having to buy the sun-scorched plastic bottles of water which are not safe for fertility.

Very often, after drinking my organic herbal tea, I will pour my water in it and use it as flavoured water all through the day and it sure has this "zing" that makes you want to drink more and more.

Makes 1 serving of a litre

Ingredients:
- *2 knobs of ginger root*

- *2 knobs of turmeric*

- *1 good slice of lemon*

- *Organic unfiltered, unheated, unpasteurized Raw Apple Cider Vinegar (ACV): I prescribe Bragg*

- *Freshly boiled water*

- Tea

Below are some precautions on choices of tea used during the fertility journey. Any of our recommended fertility-friendly herbal teas listed on our website are good to go. Unfortunately, a lot of the popular "teabags" you know are not organic and their bags are made of nylon- this means the users are consuming pesticides and plastic and these two are endocrine-disrupting. Some popular herbal teas are also not safe to use when expecting a baby. Rooibos (caffeine-free and great tea substitute), Dandelion, lemon, lemon grass, ginger, peppermint are fine. Please stay away from Raspberry, Chaste berry and anything that has caffeine (this includes your white, black, oolong, Jasmine and green teas)

Directions:
If using an infuser and loose tea- Put the sliced roots in a tea infuser and place it directly in your mug. (Instead of a

tea infuser, you can use an individual tea filter or a teapot with a filter or you can strain the roots using a sieve after the tea has steeped)

- *Wash the roots properly and scrap the outer parts and slices directly into your cup.*

- *Add two caps full of ACV*

- *Add the boiling water and allow it to steep for 10 minutes.*

Enjoy!

Go to our website to have door-step deliveries of all you need to make these cups of goodness.

Precautions When Making Ginger Tea

A cup of ginger tea can be a delicious, energizing alternative to a cup of coffee, but the most important thing to keep in mind is to drink it in moderation. For some people, that means drinking no more than one or two cups per day.

The daily maximum is considered to be 4 grams of ginger (or less than 2 tablespoons) per day from all sources including food and tea. If you have acid reflux or other conditions or are taking medication, you may need to consume less or avoid it entirely. Although ginger is said to aid digestion, drinking too much of the tea can trigger an upset stomach and loose stools in some people. Avoid drinking ginger tea before bed or at night if you have insomnia or find that it keeps you up.

Ginger may slow blood clotting, so it should be avoided at least two weeks before or after surgery and shouldn't be taken with anticoagulant or anti-platelet medications or supplements (such as warfarin, aspirin, garlic, or ginkgo) or by people with bleeding disorders.

If you have high blood pressure, gallstones, heartburn, acid reflux, or diabetes, speak to your healthcare provider before drinking it regularly. Keep in mind that ginger tea should not be used as a substitute for standard care in the treatment of a health condition.

SoPrecious Veggie Seafood Sauce

This can serve as a side/additional meal, but in the right portion & with rich seafood types, it is a full meal for me. It takes 5 major ingredients, is quite easy and will take no more than 5 minutes. Preparation saves you lots of cooking time.

Ingredients

- Cooking oil (the recommended cooking oils for optimal fertility have been listed in above chapters)

- Salt (Tread carefully in use of table salt, use sea salt preferably)

- Fresh bell pepper

- An onion (or several)

- Ugu/ Spinach /Tete/ Water leaves / Any other variety of dark green leafy vegetable (I often advise to wash your vegetable leaves in generous amount of water uncut in deep bowl of water at least 3 times, chop in tiny bits and drain before use)

Optional Recommended Ingredients:
- Ground crayfish

- Variety of sea-food: prawns, fillets from stockfish, hake, panla and dry fish

- 2 cups fresh cleaned shrimps

- 2 cups sliced mushrooms

- 1 cup chopped tomatoes

- Organic spices

Directions
- Season the seafood with some spice and pepper-Set aside

- Take a pan & place it on a cooker on medium heat.

- Add 2-3 spoons of olive/palm oil.

- Wait for the pot to warm up a bit.

- Add ½ cup sliced onions and stir until fragrant but do not fry to burn.

- Add 1 teaspoon salt (divided), pepper and other spices.

- Stir frequently for 1 minute

- Drain water off seasoned seafood mix, add and stir.

- Add the chopped vegetables

- Stir it for one more minute and season to taste.

Your sauce is ready to serve. Bon Appétit!

If you would like to have some liquid in the sauce, add from your seafood seasoning stock before adding more seasoning.

Join the exciting and engaging conversations on our social media pages and blog for more simple organic recipes for healthy fertile living.

Healthy Fats & Oil

Healthy fats and oils are pressed *(slow, low temperature & unrefined- free of chemical solvents)* expressed naturally from whole plant foods *(coconuts, nuts, seeds, avocado)* and found in wild, deep sea, short-lived fish. Healthy fats combat cellular inflammation, and improve hormonal sensitivity.

What are monounsaturated fats?
Monounsaturated fats are associated with promoting healthy cardiovascular function. They are found in natural foods such as

olive oil, nuts and seeds and their butters as well as avocados. I often hear about the buzz for evening primrose oils. Well, this oil is the worst possible oil to take for optimum egg and sperm quality as it is high in omega 6 fats and what we need to optimum egg and sperm quality are omega 3 from FISH oils (high DHA:EPA ratio is best) not seeds or plants.

Fats compete for absorption so you need to be sure that you are taking the right fats. When my clients come to me taking evening primrose oils – it is THE FIRST thing I get them to stop.

Oils

For cooking oils, choose oils that are cold-pressed, virgin and UNREFINED from the plants or seeds that they originate. The cold-press process preserves the nutritional value of the oil without using high heat or adding harsh chemicals. Be wary of oils that are industrially processed and chemically treated to extract the oils from seeds; you have lots of them in the road-side shops, malls and open markets. Their use means exposure to free radicals/toxins and damage to cellular metabolism.

Avoid oils with labels especially the term 'expeller-pressed', as it still designates that the oil has been industrially processed or expeller-pressed using friction heat & is damaged. For extreme temperature cooking, you must consider the smoke point of the oils. For this type of cooking, olive, coconut, macadamia and avocado oils are better alternatives. Avocado oil is the best oil for cooking at high temperatures, followed by macadamia oil then ghee.

All these healthy heart claims with processed "soy oil" or "vegetable oil" are propaganda. Both are predominantly polyunsaturated and chemically processed. Polyunsaturated fats are highly unstable and oxidise quickly which causes inflammation in the body. Generally, you need to stay away from food cooked in oil at high temperature because of the inflammation caused by the chemicals produced. This includes all those road-side beanballs (akara), roadside small chops and fries, shawarma, etc.

Let me clarify something about cholesterol getting heightened from food. Only 15% of total cholesterol comes from food, the other 85% is manufactured by the liver. When the cholesterol levels are high, the issue is an imbalanced cholesterol production by the liver from a food combination consumed long ago. Because the role of the liver in reproduction is very key, the SoPrecious7dayFertilityChallenge makes all the difference if implementation is followed religiously.

Use link below to see the various oils and smoke points for more informed decisions.

https://www.jonbarron.org/diet-and-nutrition/healthiest-cooking-oil-chart-smoke-points

All unsaturated seeds are VERY fragile and easily damaged by heat (anything over 35 degrees), light and oxygen. Use these oils for dressings or garnishes (Cold use only). Below are examples of some cold-pressed oils you can use for your meals:

- Cold-pressed Extra-Virgin Olive Oil

- Unrefined Sesame Oil

- Cold-pressed Flaxseed

- Hempseed Oil

- Unrefined or Cold-pressed Black Currant

- Avocado or Hazelnut all

The best fish oil (omega-3) supplement is one that uses anchovies and sardines. Oil from fish contains eicosapenaenoic acid (EPA) and docosahexaenoic acid (DHA); both are omega-3 fatty acids, which have anti-inflammatory activity.

The omega-3 fatty acids in fish oil help to balance the over abundance of omega-6 fatty acids found in most of our diets. When these two groups of fatty acids are out of balance, the body releases chemicals that promote inflammation. People appear to produce more of these inflammatory chemicals when experiencing psychological stress. With a fatty acid imbalance, inflammatory response to stress appears to be amplified. Prostaglandins are hormone-like substances produced within the body that regulate dilation of blood vessels, inflammatory response, and other critical processes. Omega-3 fatty acids are needed for prostaglandin formation. EPA and DHA also modulate immune function, perhaps as a result of their effect on prostaglandin production.

Essential Oils
As raw materials to my home made cleaning and personal

hygiene products, I use the essential oils that professional aromatherapists use. If you must use essential oils, I recommend 100% pure essential oils. You can diffuse them for all sorts of health benefits as well as for their pleasant aroma, and you can make your own non-toxic air-fresheners with them! (See how to make simple home-made cleaning and personal hygiene products from our blog using your everyday pantry items)

Even if the oil is 100% pure and unadulterated, I do not recommend the ingestion of essential oils because there is likelihood of toxicity even in small doses. I understand that when one is desperate for a child, there's the tendency to fall victim of information overdose, particularly via the internet. However, please be careful with taking advice from forums online. There are tons of unproven information on how solely applying some oils gets one pregnant; this is something I strongly discourage in practice. Even though I find essential oils to be useful support to fertility treatments, I do not recommend total reliance on them to get the results we help couples achieve.

Below is a list of those that are harmful to your fertility goals:

- Anise star
- Aniseed
- Basil
- Camphor
- Cinnamon
- Clary sage*

- Clove
- Cumin
- Fennel
- Hyssop
- Mugwort
- Oregano
- Parsley seed or leaf
- Pennyroyal
- Sage
- Savoury

Saturated Fats

You can eat small amounts of saturated fats from pasture-raised meat. Studies have shown that exclusively grass fed animals have significant levels of Omega 3 fatty acids. Organic butter is another healthful fat. Margarine is not recommended. Even if the margarine is made with *good oils'* and is nonhydrogenated, it tends to have artificial ingredients. Nut and seed butters are excellent as well as nutritious spreads such as hummus, pesto, tapenade and some locally made ones. Avoid buying foods containing hydrogenated fats, partially hydrogenated fats, shortening or that have mono or diglycerides on the list of ingredients.

The Nurses' Health Study looked for connections between dietary fats and fertility from a number of different angles. Among the 18,555 women in the study, the total amount of fat, cholesterol, saturated fat, or monounsaturated fats in the diet wasn't connected with ovulatory infertility. *What they did find, however, was the largest decline in fertility in women who ate transfats.*

High Quality Dairy and Iron-Rich Foods

Small amounts of full fat (non-homogenized) dairy products – particularly live culture plain yogurt are associated with increased fertility. A diet rich in iron that comes from vegetables and supplements may lower the risk of ovulatory infertility, according to results from The Nurses' Health Study II, which followed 18,500 female nurses trying to get pregnant. Ovulatory infertility affects 25 percent of infertile couples. Vegetarian foods with iron include all types of beans, eggs, lentils, spinach, fortified cereals, long-grain enriched rice and whole grains. Add vitamin C from citrus fruits, bell peppers or berries to your meals to enhance iron absorption. High iron foods include naturally dried fruits like groundnuts, cashew nuts, our local green leaf vegetables, chickpeas, adzuki beans, lentils, quinoa, kale, broccoli, molasses and organic red meats. You can boost your intake of dietary iron by using iron fortified foods such as enriched grain products (for example a high fibre enriched bran cereal with a low GI)You can help your body absorb iron by eating vitamin C rich foods (orange, kiwi, lemon, guava, grapefruit, and vegetables such as broccoli, cauliflower) at the same time as vegetable sources of iron. Use foods that are leavened, sprouted, soaked, fermented and roasted to increase the bioavailability of the iron.

The Glycemic Index

Don't get too lost in the glycemic index. The important part is to focus on eating more legumes, whole grains and vegetables in place of fruit, juice or processed grains (small chops, pastries, breads, muffins, cakes, cookies). You can improve ovulation with a diet based on at least 60% of calories from slow carbohydrates such as whole grains, dried beans and peas, vegetables and whole non-sweet fresh fruits. Avoid high GI vegetables and limit your fruit to 2 pieces a day. If you have insulin resistance, diabetes or have difficulty losing weight, the best number might be 0.

Dried fruit and vegetables aren't great for optimal fertility because they are never 100% dry and therefore will grow mould, bacteria and yeast, all of which can have a negative impact on fertility. Eat mostly low and medium GI foods, and avoid those foods with a high GI. Examples of foods with Low GI are Sweet potato Oat bran, Lentils/kidney/ Chickpeas, Quinoa, Whole milk Yogurt, Purple Potatoes, Brown/ Basmati rice, steel cut oatmeal. The Research Article Open Access article on the Glycemic Index of Selected Nigerian Foods for Apparently Healthy People revealed the result of the mineral analysis of beans consumption: Moinmoin & Beans served with stew had the highest iron and zinc contents respectively while Akara had the lowest content for both minerals. The Glycemic Index (GI) of beans served with stew was 56, Akara was 44, Moinmoin was 41 while Ofuloju was 54. The conclusion of the GI results revealed that bean products should be consumed with restriction.

Tips:

The GI of a meal can be lowered by adding:

- lemon juice or vinegar (eg add broccoli with freshly squeezed lemon juice as a salad dressing to a meal with high or medium GI foods i.e. brown rice/Wheat pasta)

- healthy fats like olive oil, walnut oil or organic butter to steam foods

- mixing low GI food with a medium/high GI food (eg beans and brown/ basmati rice)

Money Saver Tip

*Managing temperature-diets at seasons:
I slightly steam my veggies before
juicing them to make them warmer.*

*Drink hot herbal tea before meals if you
need to eat things like cold salads, etc.*

||||||||||||||||||||||||||||||||||||||||||||||||||||||||||||||||||||||||||||||

CHAPTER 8

"Identify the culprit, accept the dare for change & your miracle is close"

- Chika Samuels

||||||||||||||||||||||||||||||||||||||||||||||||||||||||||||||||||||||||||||||

The Culprits

Dairy

The Association of Earth Prospective Study Cohort's study about protein intake (amount and type) with ovarian antral follicle counts among infertile women revealed that higher dairy protein intake was associated with lower antral follicle counts in an infertile population and no intake dairy food intake is associated with reproductive hormones and sporadic anovulation among healthy pre-menopausal women. The study showed associations between increasing dairy food and nutrient intakes and decreasing estradiol concentrations as well as between cream and yogurt intakes and the risk of sporadic anovulation (sorry guys, even your Greek yogurt counts). These results highlight the potential role of dairy in reproductive function in healthy women. (US National Library of Medicine, National Institute of Health)[17]

The Harvard Nurses' Health Study found that women who ate low fat dairy products were less likely to get pregnant. The study showed that eating "full fat" dairy products, on the other hand, was associated with an increased chance of getting pregnant. This led researchers to recommend that if women are including dairy in their diet, they should consume moderate amounts of whole fat rather than low fat dairy products. However, if you have a diagnosis of endometriosis, I advise that you eliminate dairy from your diet completely. Some research has shown that dairy products may increase prostaglandins, which stimulate oestrogen. Oestrogen is responsible for common endometrial symptoms such as painful menstrual cramps, as well as menorrhagia (heavy menses), diarrhoea, nausea and vomiting.

Gluten
Celiac disease is an autoimmune disease where the small intestines are damaged by gluten. When left untreated, celiac can cause nutritional deficiencies and seriously compromise a person's health. In a recent study, a gluten-free diet did seem to improve the male partner's fertility in a measurable way, bringing his sperm morphology (sperm shape) numbers to normal.

---

17. https://www.ncbi.nlm.nih.gov/pmc/articles/PMC3644863/

Beverages

There has been some emailed questions on hot drinks so here are the guidelines for you. First feel free to enjoy them as long as they are caffeine free, preferably organic (chemical free), dairy free and soy free and no milks from long life tetra packs (lined with plastic and highly processed liquids). So what do you have then?

Like coffee? Try teechino or dandelion beverages

Like regular tea? Try rooibos

Like herbal tea? Try anything but not green tea or matcha powders (has caffeine) and buy organic tea bags not made from plastic, or even better loose leaf tea (much cheaper!)

Like milk? - make your own nut or seed milks. The popular coconut + tigernut+ ginger combination is your go to for milk substitutes.

Like chai? Make your own blend half spices, half loose leaf rooibos tea. Chai Walli is an Aussie brand that does a straight spice mix to make this easier.

Fancy something different? Try our SoPrecious golden milk. Visit our blog for loads of recipes.

Transfats

Trans fats are artificial fats that cause damage to cells and contribute to inflammation and disease. Findings from the Nurses' Health Study indicate that trans fats are a powerful deterrent to ovulation and conception. Eating less of this artificial fat can improve fertility and can also mean an increase in healthful unsaturated fats, which can boost fertility even further. The largest decline in fertility among the nurses was seen when trans fats were eaten instead of monounsaturated fats. What are trans fats? Trans fats are synthetic fats made by hydrogenation of oils. Trans fats cause inflammation in the body, thus decreasing immune function and increasing plaque build up in the arteries. The National Academy of Sciences recommends that there is no safe level of trans fats, however the average fast food eater consumes approximately 22gm of trans fats each day through processed & packaged foods.

Increasingly, studies are showing that adulterated foods (like trans fats) have unintended health consequences. You can minimize your intake of trans fats by avoiding foods with hydrogenated or partially hydrogenated fats or shortening on the list of ingredients and minimizing your intake of fast and processed foods. Trans fats are only made via hydrogenation, which is a chemical based process in a factory making liquid fats firm e.g. think canola oil turned into margarine. Any fats may be damaged if there is too much heat applied but it won't be turned into trans fats per se – however, we still want to avoid damaged fats! Olive oil will be fine up to around 180 degrees Celsius so it's perfect for baking and gentle sautéing. Just don't fry with it. Avocado is the best for high temperature cooking, as its smoke point is well into the 200s in Celsius. Macadamia oil, ghee, tallow are also great cooking oils with higher smoke points.

High Fructose Corn Syrup (HFCS)

Developed in the 80's, it involves a complex chemical process that turns cornstarch into fructose. This processed fructose, unlike glucose, can only be broken down by the liver and causes cellular inflammation and oxidative damage to the body and is linked to hyperinsulinemia, obesity, insulin resistance and mineral deficiency – all which can negatively impact fertility. HFCS (also seen on labels as glucose/fructose) – like trans fats – are found in a wide variety of processed and fast foods, including sweetened beverages.

On the other hand, a diet that is high in antioxidants, essential fatty acids and fibre acts to support our cells to remain vibrant and healthy. The anti-inflammatory diet for health is actually the same as the Mediterranean diet which has been proven to be associated with lower risk of disease. Study after study has shown that inflammation is at the root of PCOS, endometriosis and infertility, even male infertility. Avoid the following foods, ingredients and chemicals that increase inflammation and oxidative stress:

- Refined, processed foods and fast food

- Flour and products made with flour (bread, scones, muffins, pancakes, cookies, etc). -Moderate and high GI foods (white bread, bagels, crackers, refined cereals, juice, etc).

- High AGE foods such as fatty meats cooked on high heats and highly processed foods. AGE (advanced glycolation end products) is created when sugars and proteins are heated (e.g. sweet marinade on barbequed meat).

• Corn, safflower, sunflower and soybean oils which are high in omega 6 fatty acids. The imbalance of omega 3 to omega 6 fats contributes to cellular inflammation.

• High fructose corn syrup which is a highly refined product used in soda and many processed foods.

• Trans fats found as added hydrogenated fats, partially hydrogenated fats, shortening, or mono/diglycerides.

• Fried foods

• Artificial colours, flavours, preservatives, sweeteners.

• Processed soy products (tofu, soy protein, soy milk/yogurt).

Soy

What is soy? Soy products are made from soy beans. Whole food soy products like miso, tempeh and spouted soybeans are healthy if eaten a few times a week in small amounts. If you eat tofu you should choose organic tofu (like the ones from the Northern parts of Nigeria). Soy is another hormone disrupter. If you find "mixed tocopherols" while reading labels, it is indicative of soy usage. Soy needs to be 100% avoided while on a fertility journey. That is obviously in its main forms such as soy milk and as a protein substitute, but it is a sneaky ingredient and you also need to check ingredients on packaged foods, personal care products, even candles as it is often an additive.

Tofu is fresh soy bean curd, which is a quick-to-prepare source of protein that takes on the flavour of whatever you are cooking. Natto is fermented soybeans. Miso, tempeh, and seiten are fermented soybean products that have a similar taste and texture to cooked chicken. Daily consumption of *processed* soy products may have a negative impact on your fertility. We consume large qualities of processed soy products in soy milk, soy protein powders, soy "meat" products, and soy fillers. The result is that we are eating highly processed food products rather than a whole food.

Animal Protein

Small amounts of organic animal protein can be part of a healthful fertility diet. If you choose to eat red meats, choose grass or pasture-fed meat. Keep your serving size to no more than the size of the palm of your hand. It's all about portioning! Organic turkey and chicken are great sources of lean protein, especially when eaten without the skin. Use lean cuts of meat and skinless poultry. Organic eggs are an easy to digest, inexpensive source of high quality protein. You can enjoy 3 – 5 eggs a week, even if your cholesterol is high.

Short lived, deep fish such as lady fish, kote (Horse Mackerel), croaker, titus, mackerel (titus, ask for "original titus- kampala titus"), trout, herring (shawa), sardines and wild salmon are all rich in omega-3 fatty acids shown to support healthy cells and immune function, manage weight and hormone balance and reduce pain associated with endometriosis. Eliminate use of frozen poultry or foods.

Mercury in Fish

Mercury is a neurotoxin, which can damage a developing brain. Fish that is high in mercury tends to be larger fish such as tuna, swordfish, shark, marlin, orange roughy, and escolar. Limit your intake of these fishes. Instead choose short lived deep sea Pacific fishes such as wild salmon, mackerel, sardines and halibut. Choose only high quality supplements that are from 'safer' fish.

Environmental Toxins

Here, we will be discussing the ways in which your personal environment might be keeping you infertile. According to the Consumer Protection Agency in the United States – of the chemicals commonly found in our homes because we import most of our household products from the USA, at least 150 of them have been linked to infertility, birth defects, allergies, cancer, and psychological disorders. Most of the active ingredients of the locally made ones are more toxic and surely for us, the number grows exponentially daily and it's a real, yet often hidden and unknown danger in our own homes, which we must learn to protect ourselves and our families from because our fertility, health and well being are all at stake. The dangers and exposure to these Endocrine-Disrupting Chemicals – through direct contact, drinking unfiltered water, ingesting tainted and processed food, and even just breathing polluted air – impacts fertility on multiple levels. In our online blog, there is a good read that exposes 7 key fertility poisons you must become aware of, if you want to transform your fertility results. Although it's impossible to completely avoid endocrine disruptors, there is a WHOLE lot you can do to dramatically decrease you and your partner's exposure in your own home.

First, below are some actions you need to take and items to budget for replacement

- Go through your home room by room and get rid of toxic chemicals.

- Do not use plastic wrap on hot foods or place plastic wraps over food

- Do not use synthetic or toxic cleaning products (replace with natural products, Visit our website to read how you can make your own natural personal products & my recommended list of organic personal product brands)

- Do not use synthetic shampoos, soaps, creams, cosmetics (replace with natural organic products)

- Do not use plastic storage containers for food (replace with glass or stainless steel) Do not use dryer sheets

- Unfiltered water: Get a water filter unit

Impact of Cosmetics on your Fertility
Cosmetic products contain various chemical substances

that may be potential carcinogens and endocrine disruptors. Women's changes in cosmetics use during pregnancy and their risk perception of these products have not been extensively investigated. Controlling your environment is part of this partnership. Remember, this isn't a sprint. You are in competition with no one but yourself; it's okay to take the time to do make those changes but let each day meet you better and more fertile.

Download a free copy of the SoPrecious chemical cheat sheet from our website that lists a whole bunch of ingredients that are commonly in personal care and household products. The ewg.org/skindeep website is great for you to scan ingredients on. You have to search ingredients on these websites as the cosmetic brand ratings are not accurate. Eg a brand may get a rating of 1 but when you search each of the ingredients in that product on the ewg website, you may find that some of them are a 3 or a 6 which is not what you want.

It takes time but you eventually get to know the "nasties" and know what to look for. Use the *SoPrecious cheat sheet of chemicals to avoid* to get you started. Here's the trick – if you find one nasty ingredient, you may need to get rid of the product because it doesn't matter if all the rest of the ingredients are fine. What this is saying is that the rating changes depending on the different types of ingredients that it interacts with in a formula and the actual amount of the ingredient (irrespective of ingredient concentration) in the actual formula.

There is also an amazing app called "Think Dirty". You use it to scan the barcode of the product and it tells you how toxic it is. Unfortunately, it doesn't have every product on that, but it has a good number of them! Chemical Maze is another great app too. Below are products I have found safe with these websites and apps:

- Dr Bronners range of soaps, body wash, toothpastes.

- Products from poosh website.

You'll find that as your diet improves and you remove chemicals from your life, your body odour will change and you won't need to cover any smell using a fragrance. I live in a tropical climate and rarely use deodorants (and believe me, my family would tell me if I needed one). You can use original essential oils in glass for fragrance as well.

Reading the labels- Smart ways to avoid wasting money on the fertility nasties on the mall shelves

Don't believe the packaging! Packaging on products is there solely to make you buy, not inform you. The words 'organic' and 'natural' are unregulated words especially in developing countries and can be used in advertising by anyone (certified organic is different but remember one certified organic ingredient doesn't mean its fertility friendly).

Always flip the product around and read the ingredients and make sure it's the full list of ingredients not just the 'key ingredients' or 'active ingredients'.

We understand that finding new products to replace your toxic ones can be a time consuming (and sometimes frustrating) process and we would love to be able to give you a shortcut, but as with so many things in life, there is no shortcut. In the beginning, you will need to put in the time to become familiar with what ingredients are okay and which aren't. It does get easier, I promise.

So because we want to make sure you can do this and you are able to make informed decisions, here are some things that can help:

1. Download the "SoPrecious chemicals to avoid cheatsheet". This is not a finite list of ingredients to avoid but it's a great place to start becoming aware.

2. Use apps to scan product chemical status

3. Save yourself time at the shops and research product ingredients at home on their websites.

4. Constantly check the ingredients of the products you use as companies change formulations all the time and don't inform consumers. If a product has 15 ingredients and the third one you look up is on the avoid list or rates higher than a 2 on the EWG, stop checking its ingredients and move onto the next product because it doesn't matter if the other ingredients are okay.

Plastics

Plastics are prevalent in our society. While it's almost impossible to be plastic-free, your focus should be to prevent the chemicals leeching into your food. The chemicals that make up plastic are endocrine disrupters and dramatically impact fertility negatively – as well as the ability to keep a healthy pregnancy to term; (increasing) miscarriage risk also. PLASTICS are the DEVIL when it comes to optimum fertility and they are EVERYWHERE, even in forms you don't / can't recognise. (and "BPA-free" is even WORSE than the variety that contains BPA).

So, what does this mean? All plastic is toxic. There is no such thing as safe plastic. AVOID IT like the plague in the places where you KNOW and CAN. Plastic lids like on Pyrex glass containers are fine as long as the food doesn't touch and also make sure your food is cool before putting the plastic lid on. If you can avoid buying anything in plastic, do so. Buy things like nuts in bulk where you can bring your own containers. If you can avoid using frozen veggies, please by all means, do. Plastic is everywhere, so you want to avoid or reduce your interaction with it where possible. Transfer anything that does come in plastic to a non-plastic container to store in your home. Choose glass or stainless steel blenders/ drinking cups. For storage containers, pyrex containers are great and although they have a plastic lid, it is certainly a great reduction. Stainless steel is great too for dry foods. Stainless steel containers by Thermos and glass containers from Ikea (plastic lid though) as well as Klean Kanteen products can help. You may have to budget for these changes, but don't procrastinate. Making little changes here and there will add up and become great change.

When buying something that is plastic, looking at its longevity is the key – for example, a computer mouse is made of plastic but it is something that lasts for ages so it's not really a problem. Single-use plastic bags on the other hand are an environmental nightmare and you should not have your ready-to-eat food around it. For food wrapped in plastic- avoid where possible. If it is unavoidable, then unwrap and wash as soon as you get home or in the case of meat, put in another container. The same advice applies for the plastic Ziploc bags. Here is the focus, you are trying to eliminate (at least in the pre-conception and TTC phases) anything that may have hormone disrupters in it and plastic is a big culprit.

Pesticides and Cleaning Chemicals

According to the Environmental Protection Agency, over 80,000 biologically poisonous, practically indestructible chemicals have been developed and introduced into human contact in the last 50 years. Research shows that direct or residue exposure to synthetic chemicals such as those found in pesticides can temporarily and even permanently disrupt endocrine function, which is responsible for hormonal balance, optimum fertility (in men and women) as well as normal baby development in the womb and during early childhood (when kids are most vulnerable). Such chemicals are capable of damaging general health (and fertility) throughout life.

Microwaves

These fast helpers are terrible for health, and also your fertility. As with all electrical devices, they emit EMF both when in use and when not in use and plugged in. Microwaves also emit radiation when in use. What happens when you microwave your food is that this equipment messes it up at a molecular level so that basically you are ingesting warped food. This makes it hard for your body to extract the nutrients it needs because the cells of the meal have been fundamentally changed and the body has a hard time recognizing what it is. I personally like steaming food to reheat as it tastes just like it's been cooked or preheat at home before going to work and put in a thermos or just eat room temperature food.

Money Saver Tip

Eating healthy everyday is cost-effective when strict budgeting and proactive planning comes to play. Have your shopping list of "culprit replacements" so when extra money comes in as the budget permits, the money is rightly directed. If alternatives become expensive, simply live without them. For example, who says you can not live without "swallow"? Simply make your soup rich and thick, you will not need swallow and with time, your digestive system will adjust"

II

"The laws of motion were not discovered
by the contemplation of inertia"

-*Chika Samuels*

IIIIIIIIIIIIIIIIIIIIIIIIIIIIIIIIIIIIIIIIIIIIIIIIIIIIIIIIIIIIIIIIIIIIIIIIIIIIII

Fertility Illnesses in Women

1. Ovulatory Disorders

Also known as ovarian-factor infertility, these are among the most common causes of infertility. Irregular or abnormal ovulation accounts for approximately 25% – although some estimates place it as high as 33% – of all female infertility cases. The primary function of the ovary – ovulation – is tightly regulated by hormones. So anything that throws off a woman's hormones can cause ovulatory problems and miscarriages.

Amenorrhea (total absence of menstruation), continuous menstruation, and abnormal periods – such as heavy flow, cramps, or irregular cycles – can all be symptoms of ovulatory dysfunction. Certain lifestyle factors – such as being under- or overweight, excessive drinking, or the use of certain drugs – can interfere with ovulation. They can cause progesterone defects, which are one of the most common ovulation problems and among the most common causes of anovulation. Other possible causes include any impairment in hypothalamic, pituitary, or ovarian function – such as hyper- and hypothyroidism or diabetes – which can lead to irregular or total absence of ovulation. Indeed, uncontrolled diabetes can cause both infertility and pregnancy loss.

2. Polycystic ovarian syndrome (PCOS or PCOD):

This is a hormonal abnormality that typically starts around puberty and causes ovulatory problems. It is also known as SteinLeventhal Syndrome or hyperandrogenism. This abnormality – which affects about 5 percent of all women – causes the woman's ovaries to produce an excess of androgens, the male hormones. The ovaries then develop an excess of immature egg follicles or cysts and become enlarged. Polycystic ovary syndrome (PCOS) is recognized as the most common endocrine disorder of reproductive-aged women around the world. Women with infertility related to polycystic ovarian syndrome (PCOS) do appear more likely to develop cardiovascular disease and metabolic disorders such as diabetes than the general population.[18] PCOS causes irregular or anovulatory menstrual cycles, and, as a result, infertility. Women with PCOS also commonly suffer from obesity, severe acne, hirsutism – abnormal hair growth on the face, chest, upper arms, legs, and back, which gives them a masculine look.

---

18. *https://www.ncbi.nlm.nih.gov/pmc/articles/PMC5306404/*

Polycystic ovary syndrome (PCOS) is the most common cause of anovulatory infertility in women of reproductive age. A lifestyle change is considered the first line intervention for the management of infertile anovulatory women with PCOS, and weight loss for those who are overweight or obese. Polycystic ovary syndrome (PCOS) is complex with reproductive, metabolic and psychological features. Infertility is a prevalent presenting feature of PCOS with approximately 75% of these women suffering infertility due to anovulation, making PCOS by far the most common cause of anovulatory infertility. Evidence was synthesized and we made recommendations across the definition of PCOS including hyperandrogenism, menstrual cycle regulation and ovarian assessment. Approximately 80% of women who suffer from anovulatory infertility have PCOS. Lifestyle intervention is recommended first in women who are obese largely on the basis of general health benefits.

It affects women across their reproductive lifespan and is associated with pregnancy complications, including gestational diabetes, preeclampsia, and large gestational-age babies. PCOS is associated with excess weight gain, which, in turn, exacerbates the health burden. Therefore, weight management, including a modest weight loss, maintenance of weight loss, prevention of weight gain, and prevention of excess gestational weight gain, is a first-line intervention for women with PCOS during and independent of pregnancy.

Outcomes of weight management programmes in women with PCOS are likely to be improved with the inclusion of behavioural and psychological strategies, including goal setting, self-monitoring, cognitive restructuring, problem solving, and relapse prevention.

Strategies targeting improved motivation, social support, and psychological well-being are also important. These are applied to our intervention management cycles at different reproductive life stages. Weight loss is the primary therapy in PCOS-reduction in weight of as little as 5% can restore regular menses and improve response to ovulation- inducing and fertility medications.

PCOS women can have difficulty conceiving. Those who become pregnant are at risk for gestational diabetes (which should be evaluated and managed appropriately) and the microvascular complications of diabetes. Assessment of a woman with PCOS for infertility involves evaluating for preconceptional issues that may affect response to therapy or lead to adverse pregnancy outcomes and evaluating the couple for other common infertility issues that may affect the choice of therapy, such as a semen analysis. Women with PCOS have multiple factors that may lead to an elevated risk of pregnancy, including a high prevalence of IGT—a clear risk factor for gestational diabetes—and MetS with hypertension, which increases the risk for pre-eclampsia and placental abruption. Women should be screened and treated for hypertension and diabetes prior to attempting conception. Women should be counseled about weight loss prior to attempting conception. Lifestyle interventions to reduce weight in obese women with PCOS are even more important than in obese women without PCOS.[19]

3. Hyperprolactinemia
An excess of the hormone prolactin is another hormonal imbalance

19. *American Association of Clinical Endocrinologists, American College of Endocrinology, and Androgen Excess and PCOS Society Disease State Clinical Review: Guide to the Best Practices in the Evaluation and Treatment of Polycystic Ovary Syndrome - Part 2. Https://www.Ncbi.Nlm.Nih.Gov/pubmed/26642102*

that often leads to fertility problems in both women and men. Prolactin– which is secreted by the pituitary gland–increases during pregnancy and is responsible for milk production after childbirth. One of the symptoms is galactorrhea, the abnormal production of milk in women who aren't pregnant.

4. Fibroids

Fibroids are present in 5-10% of infertile patients, and may be the sole cause of infertility in 1-2.4%, fibroids may also compromise fertility by altering the endometrial receptivity (14, 15); thus negatively affecting embryo implantation and lowering the chances for pregnancy. Fibroid location is of critical importance in ART outcomes.[20]The fact that a woman has fibroids does not mean she cannot get pregnant. One of the myths I often hear is that the presence of fibroid means the woman will most likely not carry to term and even if she does, she will most likely give birth through a caesarean section. Well, at least, I busted that myth; one of my critical factors preventing pregnancy was multiple fibroids and I carried my baby till term and had a vaginal birth. The risk of developing complications during pregnancy increases if the fibroids are over 3 cm in size. However, women with fibroids larger than 10 cm can achieve vaginal delivery approximately 70% of the time (Obstetric outcomes in women with sonographically identified uterine leiomyomata.[21]

In our fertility interventions, we have our partner fertility medical practitioners evaluate clients via pelvic exam and ultrasound

20. *The impact of uterine leiomyomas on reproductive outcomes.*
    Cook H, Ezzati M, Segars JH, McCarthy K, Minerva Ginecol. 2010 Jun; 62(3):225-36)

21. *Qidwai GI, Caughey AB, Jacoby AF Obstet Gynecol. 2006 Feb; 107(2 Pt 1):376-82.*

to delineate the location and size of any fibroid(s). For clients pursuing assisted reproduction, a pre-conception saline infusion sonogram is recommended to identify submucosal fibroids. Once a client becomes pregnant, determining the fibroid location relative to the placenta and cervical canal may be helpful in assessing the risk of placental irregularities so that early interventions can be added.

Fibroids are abnormal growths that develop in or on a woman's uterus. Sometimes these tumours become quite large and cause severe abdominal pain and heavy periods. In other cases, they cause no signs or symptoms at all. The growths are typically benign, or non-cancerous.

There are four types of fibroid:

- **Intramural**: This is the most common type. An intramural fibroid is embedded in the muscular wall of the womb.

- **Subserosal fibroids**: These extend beyond the wall of the womb and grow within the surrounding outer uterine tissue layer. They can develop into pedunculated fibroids, where the fibroid has a stalk and can become quite large.

- **Submucosal fibroids**: This type can push into the cavity of the womb. It is usually found in the muscle beneath the inner lining of the wall.

- **Cervical fibroids**: Cervical fibroids take root in the

neck of the womb, known as the cervix.

The classification of a fibroid depends on its location in the womb. Fibroids have short and long term solutions. In the short term, surgery may be required. The long term solution involves hormonal balancing to prevent regrowth and optimise fertility. Sometimes, surgery for fibroids is unavoidable because there really isn't anything natural that will necessarily shrink fibroids. Sometimes, though, it does not matter that they are there at all. You can schedule a talk with our fertility coach for a more accurate diagnosis.

Oxidative stress or cellular inflammation

Each day, our body works to keep us healthy. We even have a built-in detox system. If we take good care of ourselves through diet, exercise, stress management and a clean environment, the body ages naturally and we retain our energy, vitality and health as we age. However, in the real world, most of us have had more than our fair share of exposure to stress, pollution, stress, medications, drugs, smoke, stress, environmental chemicals, stress, trans fats, artificial preservatives, colours and flavours. These push our natural defence system to the edge, causing oxidative stress and cellular inflammation.

Oxidative stress or cellular inflammation is the root of premature ageing and disease. It affects every cell and organ and depletes our energy and vitality. Oxidative stress is a warning sign of impending neurodegenerative disease and it makes us older than we really are. The good news is that diet plays a powerful role in promoting or preventing cellular inflammation and oxidative stress.

A diet that is high in sugar, trans fats, saturated (animal) fats, refined carbohydrates, high fructose corn syrup and artificial chemicals can actually accelerate this cellular ageing process and disease. This is what has resulted in an epidemic of diabetes, diabesity, obesity, impaired glucose tolerance, heart disease, cancer, gastrointestinal problems, autoimmune disease and food allergies.

Money Saver Tip

If you haven't gotten pregnant within six months of unprotected sexual intercourse, then the male partner should go for a semen analysis. Although this will ultimately have to be done and even repeated several times, doing it early can save time and lots of money.

CHAPTER 10

*"As an expecting or pregnant mother,
you are not just what you eat. Your
unborn children may likewise be."*

-Chika Samuels

Dietary Interventions for Fertility Illnesses

Earlier on in the chapter, I mentioned that during the critical window of time from conception through the initiation of complementary feeding, the nutrition of the mother is the nutrition of the offspring – and a mother's dietary and lifestyle choices can affect both the early health status and lifelong disease risk of the offspring. Let us have a look at some dietary interventions for popular fertility illnesses:

Anti-inflammatory and oxidative stress-reducing recommendations

Foods that score high in an antioxidant analysis called ORAC may protect cells and their components from oxidative damage, according to studies of animals and human blood at the *Agricultural Research Service's Human Nutrition Research Center on Ageing* at Tufts in Boston. ARS is the chief scientific agency of the U.S. Department of Agriculture.

ORAC, short for Oxygen Radical Absorbance Capacity, is a test tube analysis that measures the total antioxidant power of foods and other chemical substances.

High ORAC fruits and vegetables that are loaded with anti-inflammatory antioxidants.

ORAC means oxygen radical absorption capacity. It is a test tube measurement of the total amount of antioxidant activity of a particular food. The Highest ORAC foods are aecia, alfalfa, apple vinegar, applesauce, asparagus, avocado, basil, beans, beets, bell peppers, black eyed peas, black pepper, blue berry, blackberry, broccoli, Brussels sprouts, cherries, chili powder, cilantro, cinnamon, cloves, cocoa, cranberry, dates, eggplant, elderberry, figs, Fiji apples, ginger, green tea, high quality olive oil, kale, nuts, oatmeal, oranges, oregano, parsley, peaches, pears, plums, pomegranate, prunes, purple cauliflower, purple sweet potato, raisins, raspberry, red cabbage, red grapes, red leaf lettuce, red potatoes, spinach, strawberry, tangerines, and turmeric. Adding fresh and freshly dried herbs and spices can increase the antioxidant potential of the entire meal.

PCOS Dietary Intervention

Diet and lifestyle play a crucial role in treating PCOS. The goal is to regulate the blood sugar, decrease insulin resistance and improve glucose metabolism. This will help to stabilize insulin levels, moods and weight. Following our anti-inflammatory, low glycaemic diet can keep your blood sugar stable, improve insulin sensitivity, and reduce phlegm.

Here are ten tips to kickstart your SoPrecious PCOS diet:

1. Eat carbohydrates with a low Glycemic Index (GI) such as vegetables and whole grains. It is very important for women with PCOS to completely avoid refined carbohydrates including sugar, white flour, whole wheat flour and products made from them such as pasta, breads, desserts, soda, and candy.

2. Keep your blood sugar stable with a daily schedule of meals and snacks every three to five hours that includes some protein and good fats (for example some nuts/nut butter, seeds/seed butter, hard-boiled egg, hummus dip). Protein foods take up to 5 hours to digest while carbohydrate foods digest within 30 minutes.

3. Eat at least five servings a day of vegetables including two servings of leafy greens

4. Have a daily serving of legumes like black beans or lentils.

5. Enjoy grass or pasture fed meat up to three times a week

6. Eat at least three daily servings of fruits like berries, which have a lower glycemic impact. Each serving of fruit should be enjoyed as part of a meal or with a protein.

7. Limit or eliminate milk and dairy as these can aggravate internal dampness. If you do have dairy, have only non homogenized full fat milk.

8. Pay careful attention to portion sizes in order to moderate glucose load and minimize insulin resistance

9. Add one or two tablespoons of cinnamon on cereal each morning to help decrease insulin resistance.

10. Include prebiotic and probiotic foods which promote the growth of beneficial bacteria in the intestinal tract. Prebiotics are found in whole grains, onions, bananas, garlic, honey, leeks, artichokes and some fortified foods. Probiotic foods are found in fermented foods (sauerkraut, live culture yogurt, kim chi, miso).

In addition, get your heart rate up with at least 30 minutes of vigorous exercise every day. Studies have shown that exercise can reverse diabetes and improve insulin sensitivity as well as help with weight control. Just losing five to ten percent of your body weight, if you are overweight, can restore your menstrual periods and reduce distressing symptoms like facial hair and acne. However, it is important not to exercise too hard. Excessive exercise depletes your *yin(coolness/balance)* and can raise your testosterone levels. This is not the time to start marathon training. Balance is the key!

Here are some recommended supplements for PCOS

- Chlorophyll: reduces symptoms of hypoglycaemia without raising blood glucose level

- B vitamins, magnesium, alpha lipoeic acid and conjugated linoleic acid: improve insulin resistance

- N-acetylcysteine (NAC): Regulates blood sugar and is a strong anti oxidant

- Saw Plamento – blocks the production of DHT (dihydrtestosterone)

- Bitter melon and fenugreek- Regulate blood glucose

In general, lifestyle changes which include weight loss, insulin control and SoPrecious fertility intervention with herbs and acupuncture have proven to be very effective in the intervention of PCOS and stimulating ovulation.

Endometriosis

Endometriosis affects 10 to 15 percent of women between the ages of 24 and 40 years of age. The triad of symptoms include dysmenorrhea (pain during menses), dysparenunia (pain with intercourse) and infertility. Endometriosis is the growth of endometrial tissue in other areas of a woman's body besides the uterus. This tissue is usually found in the abdomen – on the ovaries, fallopian tubes, the ligaments that support the uterus, between the vagina and rectum, the outside of the uterus or the lining of the pelvic cavity – but also sometimes on the bladder, bowel, vagina, cervix and vulva; and very rarely, in the lungs, arms and legs. The cause of endometriosis is not clear, but it has been strongly linked to immune system dysfunction and exposure to dioxins and other toxic chemicals that accumulate in the fat stores of fish, animals and people.

The priority is to first minimize PCB and dioxin exposure and consumption in the home, workplace and diet. The SoPrecious one-on-one detoxification programme along with a personalised anti-inflammatory diet is recommended with an emphasis on the following:

- Eat high fibre foods which increase transit time in the intestines and promote optimal balance of probiotics in the intestines. Avoid meat because it contains large amount of arachidonic acid with promotes inflammatory prostaglandins and inflammation and pain. Increase liver friendly foods such as kale, Brussels sprouts, broccoli, rapini.

- Use more anti-inflammatory spices such as turmeric (which protects against environmental carcinogens and decreases inflammation), ginger, milk thistle seeds, and ground flaxseeds. Avoid sugar, caffeine and alcohol.

- Avoid or minimize dairy products (they cause the

lipid pathway to be tipped toward prostaglandins and leukotrience that cause inflammation and vascular constriction).

- Supplement your diet with fish oil to help to reduce pain symptoms and decrease inflammatory response. Choose only supplements from an approved source that has proven low mercury, short lived, deep water fish.

Male Infertility and Dietary Interventions

Reproductive health is the result of your body being in proper balance. Stress, a poor lifestyle, inadequate diet and other factors can disturb natural balance. This results in poor health including impaired semen quality and quantity. It takes 100 days for your body to create and mature sperm. A healthy diet and lifestyle can increase sperm production, increase the percentage of healthy sperm, and improve sperm movement. Your nutrition has a direct impact on sperm potency and motility.

Research shows that poor eating habits and regular consumption of alcohol, for instance, can lower the quality and quantity of sperm, making conception more difficult. And since infertility is nearly as much a man's issue as a woman's – up to 40% of fertility problems can be traced to men – eating healthily now will boost your chances of conceiving a child. The following diet and lifestyle changes can help with male infertility:

- Losing excess weight – weight loss can increase testosterone, energy and vitality.

- Avoid soy and soy-based products.

- Eating a balanced anti-inflammatory fertility diet to ensure maximum intake of minerals.

- Choosing organic foods and chemical free personal hygiene and cleaning products.

- Eliminating caffeine, alcohol, tobacco, and marijuana.

Eat only low mercury fish and organic meat, poultry and dairy to minimize exposure. Another slimy food that's rich in the ever-important zinc is prawns! Prawns will also help boost your immune system and increase male sex drive.

Money Saver Tip

*Do your research online before
you head to the shops.*

*Find your local health food/organic
shop online see what brands they have
and then look up the ingredients using
the SoPrecious chemical cheat sheet.*

CHAPTER 11

||||||||||||||||||||||||||||||||||||||||||||||||||||||||||||||||||||||||||||||

"Believing and living a fertility myth/lie could keep you in an endless circle of frustration"

-Chika Samuels

||||||||||||||||||||||||||||||||||||||||||||||||||||||||||||||||||||||||||||||

Fertility Misconceptions

Let's bust some myths: It's time to sort the facts from fiction. There are many myths and misconceptions you're bound to encounter during your pursuit of pregnancy. While some may have elements of truth, most ultimately don't hold up to scientific scrutiny, or are yet to be proven or disproven. Here are some popular myths about conception.

Myth 1:
The "missionary position" is best if you want to conceive.

The reality: Many people assume that if the female partner is on top during sexual intercourse, sperm will leak out of the vagina, reducing the chances for conception. However, that's not true. Somehow, the sperm manage to make it to where they need to be, whether or not the couple engages in the missionary position. The force of the ejaculation, regardless of the man's position, is enough to propel sperm into the cervical mucus. It's only the sperm that get into the cervical mucus that will pass through the cervix and enter the uterus. Whatever sperm don't reach the cervical mucus will probably be rendered useless in the vaginal environment anyway. So, use the position that's most comfortable for you. It's having sexual intercourse that's important.

Myth 2:
Having an orgasm increases a woman's chance of conceiving.

The reality: While having an orgasm increases a woman's pleasure, it's not necessary for conception; that depends on whether or not a sperm fertilizes an egg. This can happen during pleasurable sex, unwanted sex, and even no sex, as in artificial insemination and in-vitro fertilization (IVF). Although some scientists theorize that the contractions of a female orgasm may facilitate the movement of the sperm toward the Fallopian tubes, healthy sperm – the kind that are most likely to fertilize an egg – will swim there on their own. And while an orgasm is usually necessary for a man to ejaculate sperm, occasionally small amounts of sperm are released prior to ejaculation.

GETTING PREGNANT WITH EASE

Myth 3:

You should stay in bed for at least a half hour after intercourse if you want to conceive.

The reality: This is a corollary to the "missionary position" belief. Some women have been told that rushing out of bed will cause millions of sperm to flow out of the vagina. As we've mentioned, the sperm manage to get to their destination in spite of the spillage. Some doctors do, however, recommend that women do stay in bed awhile with their hips elevated on a pillow. While there doesn't appear to be any medical proof for this advice, there certainly is no harm in it. Trying to conceive can put enormous strains on a couple, so while by no means necessary, languishing in bed a bit in the afterglow of the moment is soothing. Enjoy the quiet time together.

Myth 4:

Sperm can only live for about a day.

The reality: Although many sperm live for only 24 hours, they can live for up to 72 hours in the woman's reproductive system. And in some cases, sperm have been known to have lived as long as five days!

Myth 5:

Ovulation always occurs on Day 14 of your cycle.

The reality: The day you ovulate depends on many factors, including the length of your cycle. Most women have a 28-

day cycle and tend to ovulate on the 14th day. However, many women have shorter or longer cycles and will ovulate accordingly. If a woman has a 25-day cycle, she's likely to ovulate on Day 11. If her cycle is 30 days, she'll probably ovulate on Day 16.

Myth 6:

You can conceive only one day each month – the day you ovulate.

The reality: A woman can conceive up to six days each month – five days prior to ovulation and on the day of ovulation. Conception after ovulation, however, is unlikely to occur. How to determine when you ovulate is discussed in detail in the next chapter.

Myth 7:

If you ovulate from one ovary one month, you'll ovulate from the other the next month.

The reality: Ovulation does not alternate between ovaries, but is a random event with each ovary having about a 50 percent chance of ovulating each month. Some women do, however, have a dominant ovary and will ovulate from that one more than the other.

Myth 8:
If you've been pregnant before, you'll have no trouble conceiving the second time around.

The reality: Having had a previous pregnancy – especially with your current partner – is a good sign, but it's not definitive proof of your current fertility status. A lot could have happened to you or your partner physiologically that could delay or interfere with conception. Some women develop antibodies against their partner's sperm, making another pregnancy unlikely without intervention.

If you have a different partner, it's a whole different ballgame. Having been pregnant with a previous partner in no way ensures that a woman will easily conceive with her new partner. And if a male partner impregnated his previous partner, it doesn't guarantee that he's as fertile as he was in the past.

Last but not least is perhaps the most pervasive and frustrating myth of all:

Myth 9:
"Take a vacation and you'll get pregnant" or "Relax and you'll get pregnant."

The reality: Taking a vacation can help you relax, and when you're relaxed you're more likely to want to have sex. It also affords you the time to have sex, and having sex certainly increases your chances of conceiving. But the unfortunate implication behind this myth is that you're too stressed to conceive, and therefore need to relax more. This, however, has absolutely no scientific basis. Another similar myth – "Adopt and you'll get pregnant" – has also been disproven.

Get it Done by Getting the Facts

1. An understanding of how the male and female reproductive systems work is an important part of preparing to conceive.

2. The average young, healthy couple has only a 20% chance of conceiving each month.

3. It takes approximately 72 days for sperm to be produced and matured.

4. A woman can conceive up to 6 days each month.

5. By learning the facts about getting pregnant, you can disregard the many myths and misconceptions.

The Facts

- Age and poor timing of sex are 2 factors that can slow down conception. It is recommended to have sex every second day starting 2 days before ovulation. 2 days before that, your partner needs to clear out the old sperm. When unsure of ovulation, have sex every second day in the week leading up to ovulation. It means that it is much more likely that the sperm will be there ready for when you ovulate and keep having sex every second day until you confirm that you have ovulated.

Believe it or not, some of the couples that I consult, come to me saying that they can't conceive and wondering why. Yet, when I discuss with them about how often they're having sex, the answer is once every 2 months!

- Observing changes in your cervical mucus is one of the best, easiest, and cheapest ways to pinpoint ovulation.

- A minimum of 200 million sperm per ejaculation is usually necessary for conception.

- Before going to a fertility specialist, the male partner should have a semen analysis done and the female partner should have some idea of whether or not she ovulates, and when.

Money Saver Tip

Know the truth about your health or fertility can keep you off the infertile or chronic illness loop and that can sure save your time, money and energy.

||||||||||||||||||||||||||||||||||||||||||||||||||||||||||||||||||||||||||||||||||||||||||||||||||||

CHAPTER 12

"Things in life have intelligence.
The things you would like to discontinue was programmed
into existence by you. You gave them the rights to
exist in your body by your words and way of life. You
have to use a programming to destroy them."

-Rev. (Dr) Chris Oyakhilome PhD, Dsc, D.D
||||||||||||||||||||||||||||||||||||||||||||||||||||||||||||||||||||||||||||||||||||||||||||||||||||

Spiritual Practices & Effective Mind Management

In an earlier chapter, I mentioned that our primary food comprises of healthy relationships (with self, family, and community), the right oral intakes, regular physical activity, a fulfilling career, a spiritual practice & effective mind management. Life is spiritual and that which we see in the physical is only a caricature of the spiritual. Believe it or not, everything you see with your optical eyes is "remote-controlled" from some place called the spiritual realm.

There are spiritual laws and there are physical laws and the beautiful thing about laws is that they are in action whether or not you believe they exist. For example, you will fall off the balcony if you let go and fall, irrespective of if you believe in the law of gravity or not. Some of these spiritual laws will be discussed here and these are truths that I have tried out and seen play out in my life and that of my loved ones.

Spiritual things can often be difficult to communicate, but the Bible shows that we can understand them by looking at the physical. That's because the spiritual gave birth to the physical. The bible in Hebrews 11:3 tells us, *"...the worlds were framed by the word of God, so that things which are seen were not made of things which do appear."* Those that have made a difference in their generation are the ones that took advantage of these laws and used them to produce the extraordinary in an ordinary world.

I must say that everything I will share in this chapter is wholly inspired by my life coach, mentor and the author of the book with which this subject of "mind management" has exhaustively been addressed. In this chapter, I will be sharing from the book *The Power of the Mind* by Rev.(Dr) Chris Oyakhilome, PhD, Dsc, D.D and how I adopted its principles to achieve the supernatural birth of a healthy child against the reports of world's most reputable doctors. I have read lots of articles and books on mind management but none comes close to what I learnt from this book *The Power of the Mind*. Not only were critical questions addressed, but the HOWs were also not left out.

So, let's dive right in. First, you must believe that God's greatest desire is for you to live a victorious life. However, one reason many are still struggling to live that glorious life is *their inability to appropriate to themselves what God has already made available to them*. God, in His loving-kindness has, however, equipped us with *a special instrument* to help us *appropriate and come into full possession* of these manifold blessings. **That instrument is the mind!**

In *Romans 12:2*, Paul tells us about one of the wonderful gifts, God gave us and its function; he said, **"And be not conformed to this world: but BE YE TRANSFORMED BY THE RENEWING OF YOUR MIND, that ye may prove what is that good, and acceptable, and perfect, will of God."**

This scripture was a game-changer for me. You mean that God has given us our minds for our transformation? I read that the English word *"transformed"* is from the Greek word *"metamorphoo,"* which means *"to be transfigured or changed from one form, state, or level to another."* So I believed that through my mind, I can change my "state" and "form" from barren or infertile to fertile and productive.

I read on to know that you must know *how to* use this tool called the mind. I got to understand that for my expectations to be actualized, then the content and character of my mind must be rich and positive enough to pull toward these expectations towards me. This is my responsibility, and God expects me to do it. But HOW? I read on and found that the way to transform, improve, and upgrade my life is by "renewing my mind". This spiritual principle tagged "MIND MANAGEMENT"; was rightly defined as the concept of reorganizing or reprogramming one's mind (its contents and processes) with God's Word and aligning one's thinking, perceptions and mindset about God, other people, the world, and yourself, with His Word. This definition is so full and complete- nothing missing!

You see, who you are today is a function of your mind. The Bible says as a man thinks in his heart, so is he *(Proverbs 23:7)*. Your life and the totality of your personality *(how you live, what you do, the character of your words, etc.)* are the expressions of your mind. I can easily relate to this because as I engage my clients, I can tell the state of their minds from the character of their words and shared thought processes.

 Now, God has shown you that you **can** manage your mind. That means you *can work on your mind* and change its contents, and the amazing part for me is that this change will show up in your body as conception and delivery of a healthy newborn. Managing your mind is a core part of the SoPrecious Fertility Intervention Programme because we have found that man is a spirit and if we address all physical intervention and the mind is ignored, results may elude.

Another learning point is that the mind is an intangible, spiritual entity, and only God's word can shed the best light on it. Here is a beautiful definition of the mind: **The mind is the faculty of man's reasoning and thoughts. It holds the power of the imagination, recognition, and appreciation, and is responsible for processing feelings and emotions, resulting in attitudes and actions.** There are some key words in this definition, the first of them being "thoughts."

Thought is the creation, recalling, reviewing, and processing of images, for meaning, reason, language, and expression. To me, this meant that I could create my baby, recall his image, review, and process these images for meaning. This is because you can *give meaning to the images you get*. You can also *process those images for reason, language, and expression*. All of these take place in the mind. Your mind has the ability to see, hear, perceive and interpret, even though you can't physically locate it in your body. It resides in your soul, and is a spiritual entity that only God can see.

Romans 12:1-2 tells us: **"I beseech you therefore, brethren, by the mercies of God, that ye present your bodies a living sacrifice, holy, acceptable unto God, which is your reasonable service. And be not conformed to this world: but be ye transformed by the renewing of your mind, that ye may prove what is that good, and acceptable, and perfect, will of God."** Notice he says in the first verse, "...*ye present your bodies*"; this means *you (the inward man) own your body*. He lets you know that your human spirit has power over this seeming disease-defiled infertile body.

Here is another thought: you see the words "heart," "soul," and "mind" are used interchangeably in Scripture. Let's read from the NIV translation of *Luke 24:38*

> **"Why are you troubled, and why do DOUBTS rise in your MINDS?"** (Luke 24:38 NIV).

You see, people are often afraid of what they don't understand, or things beyond their control. Doubt is preceded by fear which comes from the previous negative information received. Why do you have doubts in your hearts that this intervention may not work? This is because of information from the past: experiences, doctors' reports, words from others, etc. For a woman trying for a child for 7 years, you can be sure that there is no manner of counsel I did not receive – I shared a lot of these experiences in my free e-book which you can download on our website. I often tell people, "Your mind is not a dumpsite, you must protect it!"

This brings us to the role of community as earlier mentioned in previous chapters. The people you hang out with matter, especially when it seems like you are desperately in need of something life-changing like bringing forth a child. The advice you open yourself to can mar your future or even that of the child IF you finally bring in one by the wrong means.

If the issue was to have a child, trust me, I was spoilt for options and would not have waited that long for a child. The issue was not whether these options will not produce a child, all my friends/ colleagues/ family that used those options/ knew someone that used them had babies to show that those options were valid. The issue was that I did not just want a child, I wanted to birth a child according to the will of God (godly seed). I was not ready nor willing to bring into this world a child with the enabling tools of the evil one. Is it modern native doctors that are now on an online spree with e-commerce delivery of charms? Or the dogs in the house of God and family friends who propose to sleep with you to 'help get you pregnant' & no one will know? Or worship places that are modern day household of evil works taking advantage of desperate women to bring in demon-babies? The options you are faced with in a search for a child are endless and you must ask yourself, "WHY do I really want this baby?". So many women have allowed themselves to be a channel for breeding demon-babies and will have the rest of their lives to deal with that, because the devil gives no free gifts; this is asides the menace to society these creatures will cause.

When you leave your mind open, any worthless seed can be thrown in it and it'll grow. It's your spirit that the Bible describes as a field, not your mind. And because your spirit is only accessible through your mind – which is the door to your spirit – nothing can get in there that you don't first allow in your mind. That's why the Lord instructs us: **"Keep thy heart with all diligence; for out of it are the issues of life"** (Proverbs 4:23) I love James Moffat's delivery of Proverbs 4:23-24 "...guard your inner self so you can live and prosper. Bar out all thoughts of evil and banish wayward words." The word "guard" has a military connotation, which suggests protecting from attack or maintaining in safety from danger. There's an adversary, and that's why the Lord instructs you to keep – or guard – your heart with all diligence. If someone says something to you that challenges God's word, bar it from your mind! Don't try to accommodate it or reason it out. The Lord told us the files to delete from our minds and the new ones to download and replace them with.

"Finally, brethren, whatsoever things are TRUE, whatsoever things are HONEST, whatsoever things are JUST, whatsoever things are PURE, whatsoever things are LOVELY, whatsoever things are of GOOD

REPORT; if there be any VIRTUE, and if there be any PRAISE, think on these things"

Philippians 4:8

How remarkable this is! It immediately shows us God's yardstick for measuring good thoughts. It says whatever things are consistent with truth [God's word], excellent, lovely, of good report, and praiseworthy, focus your mind on these. In other words, let these thoughts occupy your mind and control your thinking process. So my question to you is, "What has been on your mind?" Imagine the kind of life you'd be living if this verse of scripture controlled your mind? How many times have you heard something that wasn't true, or honest, or pure, or of good report, but you kept it in your mind and thought about it?

Maybe an in-law told you hurtful words, or you ran into your classmates with their battalion of kids or you saw their posts of family vacations and it kept you up all night, musing and tossing in your bed. Are you allowing the thoughts of failed IVF and miscarriages torment you, seeing these negative images and reliving the nasty experiences again every time you close your eyes, which only serve to upset you even more? Why do you let yourself worry so? These are self-inflicted, internal conflicts that you must let go of. Why hold on to something that's a connection to unhappiness? Did you know that negative thoughts could reconstruct your face and cause you to look older? I have met with intending moms that are 32 and already look 45 and even older than their spouse.

I had a client that had diagnoses of fibroids and started accurately applying all we prescribed at our one-on-one intervention programmes and when we started dealing with mind matters, we found out that she was filling her mind with junk from all the fibroid social media pages there are. Trust me, I am for research and knowledge building but you must have a filter in your mind and seek true solutions. When the mind is filled with information about "all the things that could go wrong" and so much of "what may work", you just keep going in circles. Do you know that in the eyes of God, that fertility diagnosis or report is not true? This is because it's not in line with His provisions for you as revealed in His Word. That condition doesn't fall in line with God's definition of truth. So, refuse to dwell on it. Reject it in Jesus' name. Don't think on it, and don't voice it.

The doctor, by virtue of his training, may tell you the facts, but the Word of God is the truth *(John 17:17)*. Fact and truth are two different things. Something may have been proven or verified as a fact, but if it doesn't align with the Word of God, it is not truth. One of the first things you must learn to do with your mind is to focus it on the right thing. Isaiah 26:3 says, ***"Thou wilt keep him in perfect peace, whose mind is stayed on thee: because he trusteth in thee."*** Stop jumping from one prayer house to another, seeking for help; the helper is home in you.

Now, notice the scripture doesn't say, "...whose hands and legs are stayed on thee," but "whose mind is stayed on thee." This is very instructive. Stay your mind on God! Many parents have brought in little demons in baby-form into this world because they allowed their minds to dwell and act on evil counsel from someone whose opinion they respected. If the counsel does not measure up with God's word – I dare say it is from the pit of hell, even if the givers of the counsel are your siblings or parents. Trust me, our loved ones mean well, but they are only offering counsel from the level of knowledge they already have and this may be corrupt knowledge. The mind is so powerful; do you know that channelling your mind in a certain direction, directs energies to that matter? Many times, we underestimate the power and possibilities of our thoughts. *Until you change your thinking, you can't change your life or your current state.*

You must not be ignorant of the fact that there's an adversary (the devil), and one of the ways he'll try to sway you is by planting all kinds of wrong thoughts and pictures in your mind Thoughts like damaging words you were told while growing up, or like they say in Nigeria "your village people are after you" or that you are paying for the sins you committed years ago are some of the thoughts you must contend with. He will try to mislead you into *believing* these thoughts that can put you in the bondage of infertility for years. You may wonder, "How then can I distinguish the thoughts that come to me? How can I know the thoughts I should or shouldn't accept?" It's simple. Every thought that makes you envy a pregnant woman or those that just gave birth, or makes you work against the purposes of God, is from the devil, not from you. When you find yourself thinking thoughts that frustrate or contradict God's plans for you, or for the church, which is His Body, understand that they're not from you or God, but the devil. When such thoughts come to you, immediately discern and reject them.

While waiting for the lord for my child, I consciously ensured I bought presents for and openly celebrated it when my friends and family had babies. Every festive season, I planned children parties, food stuff and special seeds for inner city children. These were deliberate actions as I knew that as I celebrated others, soon enough, it will be my turn. Remember we defined "thought" as the creation, recalling, reviewing, and processing of images for meaning. Creating, recalling, reviewing, and processing are all up to you. It's up to you to process or not to process the images that you get. If you don't process them to have a meaning, they can't give you a meaning by themselves.

Another interesting thought from this powerful book is on *how your thoughts affect things around you*. Do you know that your thoughts can also affect your sex drive, the quality of your spouse's sperm, your ovulation, your bed, your finances? Do you know, that your room has thoughts from you? The walls, furniture, clothing, etc. in your room are made from materials that have memory and can *receive and retain* information from you, and whatever they've gotten from you can remain in them. That's because thoughts release signals, and those signals can be received by things around you and people connected to you.

You've probably had this experience where you were thinking about a particular thing and even though you hadn't said anything about it to anyone, someone near you started thinking the same thing and actually voiced that thought. When I understood telepathy, I became very careful of the thoughts I allow in my mind. If I don't want to create certain thoughts in someone near me, I won't think them, because I know I can transmit those thoughts.

Our SoPrecious fertility interventions help with easy exercises, teaching you to manage your mind. First, start learning to think happy thoughts. Practise it until you become good at it, such that whenever negative thoughts of discomfort, frustration, anger, annoyance, bitterness come to you, you can easily say no to them and change your mind. Change your thinking; start by saying the right things, uttering words of gratitude, and singing songs of praise to God.

Lets talk about "STRONG HOLDS" for a minute.

> *For the weapons of our warfare are not carnal, but mighty through God to the pulling down of strong holds;) Casting down imaginations, and every high thing that exalteth itself against the knowledge of God, and bringing into captivity every thought to the obedience of Christ;"*

> *2 Corinthians 10:4-5*

"Strongholds," in the context in which it's used above, refers to ideas, theories, imaginations, reasoning, beliefs, and so on that are contrary to God's word that attack and capture people's minds, causing them to think, act, and respond in a certain way. Strongholds are mental walls of containment that prevent people from advancing in the things of God and from enjoying their inheritance in Christ. For example, someone thinks, "I'm never going to be pregnant or deliver normally," because her grandmother and her mother had history of high blood pressure or diabetics. Another one says, "Every time I take in, all hell breaks loose and I miscarry," because that used to be her experience. These are strongholds!

Paul also talked about "every high thing": ***"Casting down imaginations, and every high thing that exalteth itself against the knowledge of God..."*** (2 Corinthians 10:5). This refers to falsely exalted systems of ethics, religion, philosophy, and so on set forth by men to oppose and defy the knowledge of God. These are vain, unfounded opinions, dogmas, mind-sets, biases, superstitions, and beliefs that have become mental barriers erected in people's minds against the knowledge of God. So, how do we pull down these strongholds standing between you and your babies?

> ***"Wherefore take unto you the whole armour of God, that ye may be able to withstand in the evil day, and having done all, to stand. Stand therefore, having your loins girt about wit truth, and having on the breastplate of righteousness; And your feet shod with the preparation of the gospel of peace; Above all, taking the shield of faith, wherewith ye shall be able to quench all the fiery darts of the wicked. And take the helmet of salvation, and the sword of the Spirit, which is the word of God:"***

Ephesians 6:13-17

Looking closely at each of these weapons, you'll observe that only one – the sword of the Spirit – is an offensive weapon; all the others are for defence against attacks. Take up your shield of faith to cover you completely, and quench all the fiery darts of the wicked one. These fiery darts are thoughts the devil fires at people's minds, and they've destroyed lives and families, ruined businesses, caused wars, and ravaged nations. With your shield of faith, you can and should quench every single dart the enemy fires at you. As you meditate on, mutter, and speak God's word, those mental barriers based on the wrong things you've heard and believed all your life will come crashing down like the walls of Jericho!

You can overthrow them all with the sword of the Spirit, and as Conybeare's translation of Ephesians 6:13 says, "... having overthrown them all...stand unshaken". I recall in my sixth year of waiting on the Lord for a child, I had tried all the principles prescribed and I was almost giving up. I went to my pastor and said, "I have tried everything in the books and yet it does not seem like my situation has changed yet." She then shared with me the scripture above in Ephesians 6:13 says, "... having overthrown them all...**stand unshaken"**

When you believe you have checked all the boxes and done all you should THEN – STAND UNSHAKEN! Do not lose faith! Do not give up, do not give in! You must also be sure that you are not "poisoning yourself", by manufacturing worry and pain. Scripture tells us in *Nehemiah 8:10:* **".... neither be ye sorry; for the joy of the LORD is your strength."** In the Hebrew text, the word translated "sorry" is "awtsab," and it means "to carve, fabricate, or fashion worry, pain, anger, displeasure, grief, hurt." So, Nehemiah was telling Israel, in essence, "Don't process, fabricate or manufacture these negative feelings and emotions of worry, pain, anger, displeasure, grief, or hurt, because the joy of the Lord is your strength."

The joy of the Lord is your strength, and God wants you to be strong in the strength He's made available to you. This is why if Satan wants you to displease God, he'll go after your joy; he'll try to stop you from being joyful and cause you to blame everybody around you for your bad feelings and emotions. If he succeeds, you'll find that you're constantly angry and upset, because someone somewhere is always offending you, hurting you, or annoying you. Then, you develop an "attitude." But what's really happening is that you're becoming weaker spiritually, because you've allowed Satan steal the joy of the Lord that should have been your strength. I see this a lot with women that are trying for children; they get angry, bitter, blaming everyone but themselves.

Like Joshua, the Lord is asking you to be strong and very courageous. If you're wondering how to be strong despite your situation, know that this strength comes from the joy of the Lord, and that joy is expressed in singing, laughter, dancing, words of praise, and the loving harmony you have with your spouse and brothers and sisters in the Lord, as you speak positive, uplifting, and encouraging words to them. Refuse to dwell on pain, displeasure, worry, and all such negative feelings and emotions. Don't set your mind on failure or on those who are trying to make trouble with you or those who laughed at you and said you will never have a child. Don't set your mind on their negative, hurtful, or hateful words. You're born of God, and you have His nature. You've been created in His image, so think and act like Him.

Be Christ-like in your attitude. Don't wait for the offender to apologise before you forgive and talk to him again. Act like God instead, Who extends His love to sinners even when they don't recognise Him. Extend your love (attention and care) to others, even if they despise and disrespect you. Give vent to the righteousness of God in your spirit, and you'll always be happy. Of course, there are people that can never be pleased. I understand that it takes two to make a relationship but "If it is possible, *as far as it depends on you*, live at peace with everyone (Romans 12:18). Do your part and move on if the other refuses to. I once had a client who just suffered miscarriage just before we met and her mind was battered, not even by the occurrence but by the emotions of those around her. I told her, "People around you may be responding negatively emotionally, but you've got to learn to respond from your spirit. God wants His Word in your spirit, and controlling your mind." The Bible says don't let anything or anyone produce the worst in you. Don't find yourself manifesting such ungodly attributes. Refuse to let your life be a vent for satanic expressions.

You don't get better by worrying. Do not worry about these things, because your Father knows you need them. Your priority should be to see God's Kingdom established and His righteousness manifested in your world. I once asked someone, "why do you want to have a child?" And she answered, "so that I can prove to my mother-in-law that I am a woman." I think that is a low-level reason to desire to bring a new life to this world. My husband and I had to ask ourselves this same question, and my response was that my inspiration for procreation is "to bless my world with an extended investment in my personality." You see, a lot has been invested in me by God, life coaches and mentors and I wanted to re-invest these rare gifts and blessings to the next generation and what better way than to use your own seed as an example to show the world how it should be done.

Before we had our baby, whenever my husband and I would go out and see a parent behaving badly towards a child or a child exhibiting the wrong traits or attitude, we remind ourselves not to judge but to have our own so we can, through that child, show how it should be done. My mother-in-law used to say that was the first sentence I learnt when I got married into their family was, "Kpe nkeyi" meaning "Judge your own, focus on your own". You see, I have come to understand that everyone is running their own race, if you have been living by rating yourself by other people's metrics, you need to take a halt and retrace your steps. You are in your own lane and you are who God says you are.

T.L. Osborn rightly said those who are concerned about what people think about them are the slaves of the last people they talked to. How true! Such people are weighed down by the burden of trying to please others. Don't strive to look good before others; be desirous to please the Lord instead. So be careful for nothing, but in everything by prayer and supplication with thanksgiving, let your request be made known unto God. Just tell Him what you want; He's big enough, and He knows everything about your life and the future. When this becomes your mindset, you'll understand that there's no use worrying about anything.

Lastly, I will share with you a spiritual principle with a guaranteed outcome. I have tried it many times and it failed not once. It is in *Philippians 4: 6-7:*

"Be careful for nothing; but in every thing by prayer
and supplication with thanksgiving let your requests

be made known unto God. And the peace of God, which passeth all understanding, shall keep your hearts and minds through Christ Jesus."

Earlier in the chapters, we talked about laws. When you understand spiritual laws and act upon them, they'll produce results just as surely as the physical laws. The principle here is that when you take no thought, but instead present your requests to the Lord in prayer and supplication with thanksgiving, the result is the peace of God protecting your heart and mind.

You may not always be responsible for how information comes to you, but you're certainly responsible for what you do with it, that is, how you process and act on it. And that's what matters. *Proverbs 4:24-25* says, *"Put away perversity from your mouth; keep corrupt talk far from your lips. Let your eyes look straight ahead, fix your gaze directly before you."* "Perversity" here refers to deviation. So, in other words, "Don't deviate in your speech or talk; Don't say affirm your bright future today and uproot the word-seeds with the wrong affirmation tomorrow, let your eyes look straight on. When God has given you His Word about your life – your work, family, marriage, children, finances, or whatever it is – don't lose His direction. Don't say the wrong things or speak outside of what God has said concerning you. Speak His word and look straight on.

There is surely light at the end of this tunnel and you are closer to it than when you began.

Get your copy of this amazing book- The Power of your Mind at https://www.loveworldbooks.org/lwb/index.php/christian-books/christian-life-living/item/the-power-of-your-mind

I had no idea how many men and women needed to hear my story until I started telling it. There is so much beyond this book that I would love to share to inspire other people all around the world. Keep in touch through our social media platforms, Don't be a stranger; join our engaging exciting community of men and women making a huge difference all around the world.

Has this book made any difference or helped you in any way? Do send us a message: *info@soprecious.ng*

How you can reach us:

Fertility issues are client-specific and so are our intervention-approach for each intending parent.

At SoPrecious Fertility/Lifestyle Intervention Centers, we offer:

1. One-on-one focused coaching sessions

2. Group focused coaching sessions

3. Referrals for medical profiling before certain interventions like supplementation, diet planning, critical factors management techniques are engaged.

We run several programmes to get you ready for the expected intervention results like:

- 100-Day Preconception Programme

- Conception Cycle Demystified Programme

- SoPrecious sustainable lifestyle management program etc.

If you are at all concerned that you might have a fertility problem, start by making an appointment by using link on our website *(www.soprecious.ng)* or send an email to *info@ soprecious.ng* to book a session with us.

We are also on social media:

@sopreciouslifestyle on Instagram

@sopreciouslifestyle on Facebook

Email us info@soprecious.ng

Mobile: +2348062808307

Printed in Great Britain
by Amazon

21324857R00120